THE
TAPPING
DIET

A Revolutionary Approach to WEIGHT LOSS

THE
TAPPING
DIET

Discover
the Power of
EMOTIONAL
FREEDOM
TECHNIQUES
(EFT)

CAROL LOOK, LCSW, EFT Master

JILL CERRETA, MS, RD, CD

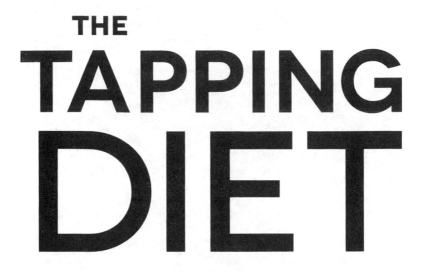

Adams media
Avon, Massachusetts

Published by
Adams Media, a division of F+W Media, Inc.
57 Littlefield Street, Avon, MA 02322. U.S.A.
www.adamsmedia.com

Contains material adapted and abridged from *Train Your Brain to Get Thin* by Melinda Boyd, MPH, MHR, RD with Michele Noonan, PhD, copyright © 2013 by F+W Media, Inc., ISBN 10 1-4405-4015-2, ISBN 13: 978-1-4405-4015-8; *365 Ways to Boost Your Metabolism* by Rachel Laferriere, MS, RD, copyright © 2010 by F+W Media, Inc., ISBN 10: 1-4405-0213-7, ISBN 13: 978-1-4405-0213-2; and *The Everything® Calorie Counting Cookbook* by Paula Conway, copyright © 2008 by F+W Media, Inc., ISBN 10 1-59869-416-2, ISBN 13: 978-1-59869-416-1.

ISBN 10: 1-4405-7911-3
ISBN 13: 978-1-4405-7911-0
eISBN 10: 1-4405-7912-1
eISBN 13: 978-1-4405-7912-7

Printed in the United States of America.

10 9 8 7 6 5 4 3 2 1

Library of Congress Cataloging-in-Publication Data

Look, Carol.
The tapping diet / Carol Look, LCSW, EFT Master.
    pages cm
Includes index.
ISBN 978-1-4405-7911-0 (hc) -- ISBN 1-4405-7911-3 (hc) -- ISBN 978-1-4405-7912-7 (ebook) -- ISBN 1-4405-7912-1 (ebook)
1. Reducing diets--Psychological aspects. 2. Weight loss--Psychological aspects. 3. Emotional Freedom Techniques. 4. Reducing diets--Recipes. I. Title.
    RM222.2.L574 2014
    613.2'5--dc23
                            2014026571

Cover design by Sylvia McArdle.
Cover image © limbi007/123RF.

This book is available at quantity discounts for bulk purchases.
For information, please call 1-800-289-0963.

ACKNOWLEDGMENTS

I would like to acknowledge the groundbreaking work of Dr. Roger Callahan who introduced the original tapping method—Thought Field Therapy (TFT)—into the field of psychology. While Dr. Callahan passed away in 2013, he forever changed the way emotional conflicts and distress are handled in the field of psychology. Without his dedication and teachings, we would not have had the level of emotional healing we now have in the world.

I would also like to acknowledge and thank Gary Craig who created Emotional Freedom Techniques (EFT), which is based upon TFT. Gary taught thousands of us how to use tapping on clients in ways that transformed their lives as well as ours. I will always be grateful for his influence and skill, and how he could see the possibility for healing in anyone.

I would also like to thank Dr. Patricia Carrington who introduced the Choices Method into the tapping field. She has changed my work through her insight, compassion, and friendship.

I want to thank the professional and friendly F+W Media, Inc. team and their partners who helped shape this book into what it needed to be: Maria Ribas, Tom Hardej, Jennifer Lawler, and Katie Corcoran Lytle.

And much gratitude to my "dream team" of coaches for their integrity, skill, and humor: Leslie Vellios, Lynn Rekvig, Marti Murphy, Catherine Duca, Heidi Garis, Betty Steinman, and Tina Marian. And so much gratitude to Rick Wilkes for always being available with his time, attention, and wisdom.

I am deeply grateful to my incredibly supportive family members—my husband, John; my sister, DeeDee; my niece, Eliza; and my nephew, Jackson—for their unconditional love and the immeasurable joy they have added to my life these past few years.

Finally, I would like to thank my clients and students who have touched my heart so deeply in my private practice, mentoring groups, workshops, and the Abundance Coaching Program. They have taught me so much about patience, connecting to my heart, and trusting my intuition.

CONTENTS

INTRODUCTION

I hate diets. Always have, always will. How about you?

Most diets fail because they assume that you just need to modify your portion sizes and get more exercise. What they overlook is the emotional component of overeating. Many people eat too much because they use food to calm their emotions. When you're upset or tired or lonely, you eat. Traditional diet plans don't address that problem. What you need is a program that eliminates your cravings and heals what causes you to overeat for emotional reasons. That increases your ability to stick to a healthy food plan. That makes you feel better about yourself, and actually helps you lose weight for good.

Enter *The Tapping Diet*—a "diet" that will help you feel better emotionally and physically because it offers a tool to help you stop emotional overeating, the missing piece to the weight-loss puzzle. When combined with the sensible food plan given in Part 2, this tool will help you finally be successful in your weight-loss challenge!

The tool is called tapping, a method that combines the benefits of traditional acupuncture with the insights of modern psychology to eliminate the emotional reasons you overeat. The technique uses your fingertips (instead of needles) to tap on acupuncture points throughout your body to reduce emotional stress. Research indicates that tapping calms down the fight-or-flight response, the response that all humans have when stress is introduced through thoughts, perceptions, or external circumstances. When you experience stress, you may often find yourself trying to protect yourself by using food to numb your emotions.

Unfortunately, you can't take stress out of your life. Your daily interactions with your family, your work, and the world around you will inevitably trigger this response. Fortunately, *The Tapping Diet* will teach you how to use tapping to reduce your stress; manage challenging emotions, such as food cravings, anxiety, insomnia, resentment, fear, sabotage, success blocks, and more; and increase your confidence and peace of mind so that the need for overeating unhealthy, high-calorie foods disappears. Throughout the book, you'll find detailed information on what tapping is and how to use it to lose weight, sample tapping scripts, a daily tapping plan, and case studies that give you real-life stories from my clients who have used this technique to lose weight and keep it off successfully, which is exactly what you're going to do, too.

Skeptical? I was, too . . . until I started using this technique on myself and my clients. For eighteen years I have successfully shared this message in person during workshops in France, Brussels, Canada, Ireland, England, and Australia, and through my training products in numerous other countries. I have also taught classes in more than a dozen states in the United States and run a coaching program using tapping as the primary tool. The result is the same: People feel hope, see results, and feel inspired and reinvigorated to use tapping to reach their goal weight. I continue to be enthusiastic and passionate about sharing this tool to help you feel calm and confident, so you can feel hope, see results, and be inspired to use tapping to reach and maintain your weight-loss goals. You can do it!

PART 1

INTRODUCTION TO TAPPING

In this part, we'll discuss the basics of tapping—what it is, why it works, and the step-by-step method you'll use to perform it (Chapter 1). Then, in Chapter 2, we'll dig into the reasons why traditional diets don't deliver results. We'll discuss the specific stressors and fears you may have about losing weight. This information will empower you to have the greatest success with tapping.

In Chapter 3, you'll learn the step-by-step specifics of how to use the tapping technique to help reduce emotional overeating and to create weight loss. You'll discover exercises and strategies that you can use to help deal with your emotions (instead of using food to numb them).

In Chapter 4, you'll develop a tapping plan that you can follow daily to help you lose weight and to stay on track with your new program, and you'll learn some additional strategies, such as meditation and visualization, that will help support your new emotional resilience.

Finally, Chapter 5 provides an enormous variety of sample scripts to use when you're tapping, covering a wide range of emotional issues you may be dealing with in your life.

Let's get started!

CHAPTER 1

WHAT IS TAPPING?

In this chapter, you'll learn the history of the tapping technique, which is formally known as "Emotional Freedom Techniques" or EFT. Based on the ancient practice of acupuncture, tapping combines the theories of Chinese medicine with modern psychology to create an innovative system for resolving the stress responses that can lead to all kinds of emotional and physical problems, including overeating. You'll learn not just what tapping is, but why it works.

Additionally, we'll go through the actual process of tapping step by step so that you can understand how to use the technique. It's not complicated, requiring only that you tap on various parts of the face or body as you recite affirmations and intentions, but it does require practice and an understanding of how to create the necessary affirmations and intentions. You'll find that tapping can be useful for dealing with many of the emotional and physical challenges you may be facing.

▶ THE DEVELOPMENT OF TAPPING

Tapping is formally known as "Emotional Freedom Techniques" or EFT. Created in the 1990s by Gary Craig, a personal performance coach in California, EFT is a simple technique that requires the client to focus on an emotional challenge while tapping on acupuncture points. The acupuncture points used in tapping were identified centuries ago in Chinese medicine. In traditional Chinese medicine, it is thought that one's life energy, or chi, moves through one's body through energy meridians or circuits. If the energy becomes blocked, a person can suffer physical and emotional illnesses. Symptoms such as pain, fear, cravings, or stress can be signs that there is a blockage between and among your energy meridians. Chinese medicine practitioners apply acupuncture needles to points on these meridians, and the symptoms disappear. In EFT and the tapping therapies, we use tapping with our fingertips rather than inserting needles to break up this energetic or emotional congestion.

EFT is based on the 1980s technique called Thought Field Therapy (TFT), which also uses tapping on acupuncture points. Thought Field Therapy was created by Dr. Roger Callahan, a clinical psychologist in California. EFT is a simpler version of this form of tapping. Craig, like Callahan before him, believed that when we release the blocked energy caused by our negative thoughts or emotional conflicts, our emotional and physical symptoms disappear. Recent research seems to confirm that tapping on acupuncture points relieves the classic fight-or-flight response that is triggered instantaneously when you think of something stressful, or think you are in danger.

TAKE NOTE

Dr. Roger Callahan's first successful tapping patient was "Mary," who had a water phobia. He applied the tapping to her while she brought up the fear in her mind. She quickly released her fear and went running down to the swimming pool at the hotel where they were working. When Dr. Callahan expressed alarm that Mary might jump into the pool even though she couldn't swim, she assured him that she had released her fear, not her common sense!

▶ THE TAPPING METHOD

Over the decades, the tapping therapies have been streamlined and made available to laypeople as well as practitioners at minimal cost and time investment. Many people have added their own spin on what works and what doesn't, what makes the tapping procedure faster or slower, harder or easier, for the layperson to apply. People have combined tapping with other therapies, such as cognitive behavioral therapy, basic talk therapy, hypnosis, and other energy techniques as well. But essentially, the basics of the approach have stayed the same.

1. A mental focus on a problem or distress (from the present, the past, or the future).
2. An acceptance statement that reduces emotional resistance to change.
3. Tapping on acupuncture points found on the face and body.

EFT founder Gary Craig initially called the EFT procedure a recipe with different ingredients. Over several decades, some of the more complicated ingredients of the EFT recipe have been dropped, as they were found to be no longer necessary for successful treatment. The form of tapping that is currently taught in workshops and seminars, online and through training products, is considered the short form and includes specific ingredients but not all that was originally included. It is what we will cover in this book.

How Tapping Works in a Clinical Setting

The tapping process is initiated by asking the client to "think of something stressful" or "think of how high your cravings are right now," which triggers the stress response in the brain. The client is instructed to measure how high this distress is on the 0–10 point scale, with 0 being no distress and 10 being the highest level of distress. Then the practitioner instructs the client where and how to tap on the face and body.

So, while the fight-or-flight response has been triggered in the client by asking for a stressful memory, the practitioner is simultaneously teaching the client how to tap on the acupuncture points, which seems to add a calming, soothing procedure that quiets down this response. Hence, the next time the client thinks about the distressing emotion or conflict, he or she is no longer as distressed by it. Several tapping rounds may be needed to significantly reduce the feeling or experience of stress. Some practitioners lead their clients to take the stress or upset all the way down to a 0 on the 0–10 point scale through multiple tapping rounds. Others have the client tap until she feels considerably better, even if she is not all the way down to a 0 when she thinks of the upsetting memory or feeling.

How Tapping Helps Treat Overeating

When past memories or current conversations leave us feeling anxious, hurt, guilty, or resentful, this stress response gets triggered in our brain and then in our bodies. We can't control the response because it's how we are wired. When this response is triggered, humans turn to a variety of immediate behavioral reactions—some people smoke; some people shut down; some people yell at their coworkers; and some people reach for food . . . lots of food, regardless of how hungry they are.

All of these impulsive remedies work in the moment, but obviously cause more harm down the road and never truly solve the problem. Not only are these quick fixes short-lasting; they don't teach us how to deal with stress in a way that could be beneficial in all areas of our lives. When we feel distress, we tend not to reach for a healing tool; we tend to resort to our most comforting behavior—overeating, for instance. Learning the tapping technique gives you a coping mechanism for dealing with stress—a coping mechanism that heals you rather than hurts you.

CASE STUDY

Lynn knew she used food to calm her emotions, but she never connected her daytime frustration from work with her nighttime cravings and overeating. She didn't have the time to satisfy her intense cravings while she was at work, but as soon as she got home after her long days, she would graze, overeat, snack, and munch until she couldn't fit anything else in her stomach. Once Lynn worked on her feelings that had spilled over from work—her anger at being underappreciated, her frustration with experiencing an unfair workload, and her resentment toward her colleagues—she was able to address and soothe these feelings with tapping, and her nighttime eating decreased tremendously. She finally became aware of the connection between her nighttime eating and her daytime frustrations, and her out-of-control eating subsided.

▶ TAPPING, STEP BY STEP

Tapping is a deceptively simple technique, but there are some basic, mechanical steps to follow that will dramatically increase its effectiveness, no matter who is using it. You might fear that it's too difficult or too weird for you to use—that meridians and Chinese medicine are too foreign for you—but I promise, once you learn the basic steps, you can easily follow the process and tap on yourself with impressive results. You do not need to understand the complex practice of Chinese acupuncture to use tapping effectively, but you do need to follow the basic steps, which are:

1. Choose a tapping target
2. Measure your level of distress
3. Devise and use your setup statement
4. Tap on specific acupuncture points
5. Measure your level of distress again

Let's dig into each of these steps a little more.

Choose a Tapping Target

When you apply the tapping to meridian points on the face and body, you want to make sure you're focused on a specific target: the condition you are working to heal. The best and simplest targets are the following:

- An emotion (guilt, frustration, anger, anxiety, loneliness)
- A symptom (physical symptoms or cravings)
- A belief ("Nothing works for me")
- A memory of an event (a time when you were yelled at in class)

If a target is too general, it's hard to focus in an efficient way. If you can't focus on the specific target, then measuring your response on the 0–10 point scale will be meaningless, and you won't be able to test whether the tapping is working or not. We know that tapping works beautifully well, but if you don't choose the right targets, the treatment won't be effective.

The clearest and best targets to choose are your emotions—stress, hurt, anger, fear, guilt, anxiety, or loneliness—because focusing on your emotions gets you immediately into a situation that you can measure and tap on for relief. (You can always amplify your feeling by asking yourself, "Where do I feel it in my body?")

If you choose a symptom that is bothering you as your target for tapping, you might choose something from this list:

- These intense cravings
- My throbbing headache
- The pain in my back
- My anxious heart-pounding
- My sweaty hands

All of these symptoms can indeed trigger your desire or cravings for food to distract you. Suffering from physical pain is an important reason people choose food, drugs, or alcohol for numbing. One of my clients said she overeats when she is cold and uncomfortable, the same way someone drinks an extra cup of coffee when he feels tired. It works temporarily because of the stimulating effect, but it does not technically make you feel less tired, and we all know the negative effects of long-term coffee drinking—fatigue, sleeplessness, and additional possible health consequences. The same is true of overeating to make you feel better. The effect is only temporary, and the long-term damage can be great.

TAPPING TIP

When you write down your target, be as specific as possible. "I feel so much pressure to get things done" is good, but "I feel stressed-out from the pressure I feel at work" is better. I'm sure you can understand why eating is much more appealing than worrying about the pressure, whether it comes from you or your boss. Food works because it is distracting—emotionally and physically.

Measure Your Level of Distress

Consider how much distress you feel when you think about your target. For example, suppose you've chosen the target, "I'm anxious about the meeting with my boss at work next week." When you think of the meeting at work next week, how distressed do you feel? How scared are you on the 0–10 point scale, where 10 is as frightened as possible, and 0 is not at all concerned?

TAKE NOTE

When you're measuring your level of distress, your emotion may not always be fear. If you're measuring a different type of emotion, consider 10 as the highest level of distress or anxiety you feel about your situation, or consider 10 as the highest level of the emotion you are measuring.

Are you a 6? A 10? Or only a 4? We take this measurement before and after the tapping so we can determine whether the tapping is working or not. In addition, we often forget how bad our stress was once we feel some relief, so having the "before and after" number is always a good objective measurement.

Take your measurement and write it down.

Devise and Use Your Setup Statement

The setup statement, originally created by Dr. Callahan to keep a person focused during the tapping process, includes a description of the problem combined with a simple affirmation, such as "I deeply and completely love and accept myself." While these affirmation statements have been changed over the years, the point is still the same: to help you feel better about yourself even though you have a serious problem to work on. So choose an affirmation that fits your personality and style.

A setup statement might sound like this: "Even though I feel scared about the meeting next week, I deeply and completely accept myself anyway." Or "even though I am anxious about the meeting at work, I choose to feel calm about it now."

If you choose as your target a physical symptom, such as your immediate cravings, the setup statement would sound something like this: "Even though I have these intense cravings right now, I deeply and completely love and accept myself anyway."

> ### TAKE NOTE
> The purpose of the setup phrase is to reduce your resistance and negativity, to make you truly accept yourself even if you don't like yourself very much right now.

The setup statement is deceptively simple. We can use the original phrasing as created by Dr. Roger Callahan. His setup phrase was routinely, "Even though I have this problem [fill in the blank], I deeply and completely love and accept myself." This phrase is repeated three times while you tap on the first acupuncture point in the system, the karate chop point, located at the base of your pinky finger and above your wrist, on the outside of either hand.

There have been many creative adaptations of this setup statement, but here's what you need to remember: Don't skip it! It's a critical part of the success of EFT (owning the problem and reducing resistance by accepting yourself). So if you use variations or adaptations of the original phrasing, make sure you are still combining the emotional description of the problem with an affirmation or phrase of acceptance.

Tap on Specific Acupuncture Points

Now it's time to tap on a sequence of acupuncture points while you focus on a reminder phrase. The reminder phrase is simply a code word or a literal description of your target. If we continue with the example, your reminder phrase would be "this anxiety about the meeting with my boss next week."

The sequence of tapping points is as follows:

EYEBROW POINT

This point is at the beginning of the hair of either of your eyebrows, above your nose. While there are other eyebrow points that serve as acupuncture points, for this method, stick to the beginning of one of your eyebrows.

SIDE OF EYE

This point is located on the outside corner of either eye. It is on the bone on the corner of your eye, not all the way back into your temple or hairline. You can use either side of your face.

UNDER EYE

This point is located on the bony orbit right under either of your eyes. It's above your cheekbone, below the actual eye socket.

UNDER NOSE

This point is on your upper lip, directly below your nose.

CHIN POINT

This point is above your chin and below your lower lip.

COLLARBONE

There are two collarbone points that are located below your neck, at the bottom of your clavicle, right under the deep indentation or 'u' under your throat. The easiest way to access these points is to put your hand in an outstretched palm and tap where the knot of a man's tie would be.

UNDER ARM

This point is located on either side of your body, about four inches below your armpit in your ribs. You may use either side of the body.

TOP OF THE HEAD

This point is on top of your head; you can tap around in a small circle.

Note: If you're having trouble visualizing where these acupuncture points are located, you can find detailed images online at *www.CarolLook.com.*

Measure Your Level of Distress Again

After completing the tapping on the specific acupuncture points on your face and body, you can measure your level of distress again, and continue with subsequent rounds as needed.

If your fear or worry felt as high as a 9 on the 0–10 point scale, and your first round of tapping reduced it to a 6, I highly recommend you continue tapping until the fear is nearly gone. Then you can go about your day without becoming fixated on the stressful meeting with your boss.

CHAPTER SUMMARY

In this chapter:

- We discussed the history of tapping, which is formally known as EFT ("Emotional Freedom Techniques").

- We learned how tapping combines techniques from the traditional Chinese medicine practice of acupuncture with modern psychological insights to help people calm their reactions to stress.

- We covered the basics of why the tapping method works to relieve stress and how this connects to weight loss.

- We concluded with a step-by-step walk-through of the tapping methodology so that you can practice tapping at home.

CHAPTER 2

GETTING TO THE ROOT OF THE PROBLEM

In this chapter, you'll discover why all of those diets you've tried in the past haven't helped you lose your excess weight and keep it off. If you're like most overweight adults, you've probably been discouraged by losing a little weight and then gaining it back, or losing a few pounds but reaching a plateau and not being able to lose more. Here, you'll gain a deeper understanding of why traditional dieting—whether it requires counting calories or eliminating certain foods from your kitchen entirely—doesn't work.

You'll also learn that you likely have stressors and fears related to losing weight. While you're probably positive about the idea in general—losing weight will improve your health, for example—you may also have a lot of anxiety about the issue. This is especially true if you've tried diets in the past. You may think you're just setting yourself up to fail again, and no one looks forward to feeling like a failure. We'll talk about how you can address those stressors and fears using the tapping method.

▶ WHY DIETS DON'T WORK

In spite of the billion-dollar diet industry in our economy, traditional diets rarely work. While anyone can lose a few pounds, even reach a goal weight through food management or food plans that are different, new, and restrictive, studies have shown that over the long term this approach of restricting food groups or calories has a debilitating effect that can backfire.

Everyone reading this book has tried between one and twenty fad diets. Some were probably absurd and others were perhaps quite reasonable. But why doesn't the weight stay off for more than a few weeks or months?

Diets don't target the real problem, so the results can't last.

Diets are by definition restrictive. They either restrict the calories you take in or restrict the kinds of foods you are allowed during the day. For instance, you are either limited to a 1,400-calorie diet, or you're not allowed to eat carbohydrates or sugar. This behavior of restriction actually harms us emotionally and backfires in a number of unfair ways. Just thinking about being allowed to eat certain foods and not allowed to eat others triggers the part of us that wants to rebel. We want what we want, and our good intentions of being on a diet go haywire fast when we restrict ourselves.

What scientists know is that when your body is denied enough calories to support its natural functioning, it responds by slowing down your metabolism so that you have enough calories to weather an anticipated famine. This reaction is hard-wired from our ancestry. Our bodies will protect us from starvation at all costs.

Starving isn't normal, and while many diets aren't so restrictive that you are literally starving, many of them that promise results would be considered a starvation plan by your physician. So I can't recommend enough that you be on a healthy eating plan rather than a restrictive one. (See Part 2 of this book for healthy recipes to support your weight-loss goals.)

So first, psychologically, we can't help but feel compelled to rebel and cheat on a restrictive diet. When we feel deprived, we want to get more, take more food into our bodies, and we tend to rebel and want what we can't have.

Then, biologically and physically, our bodies think we've gone into starvation mode and slow down our metabolism to conserve the few calories we have consumed. It's hard to live a normal life this way. We have families, jobs, social functions, and events to attend. Sticking to a restrictive diet can feel nearly impossible when tempting foods are in front of you. Again, a restrictive diet doesn't work because it triggers us to want to cheat on it or break it, but a healthy eating plan does work.

Most importantly, diets don't work because diets address food choices, not the *real* reason we make poor food choices in the first place. When you learn how to get to the root cause of overeating, your weight-loss plan can be successful and permanent.

▶ THE EMOTIONAL CORE OF OVEREATING

"It's not what you're eating; it's what's eating you."

This has become a popular phrase over the past few decades for people struggling with cracking the code to dietary success. And it's the right focus to uncover the real reason you are overeating. I use this principle by asking specific questions to help you get to the root of what's eating you:

- Why are you so hungry?
- What are you hungry for?

When you really think about it, it doesn't make sense to keep eating and eating when you're not truly hungry. That would be like filling your gas tank up and then taking the nozzle and filling up the trunk of your car, too. You don't need the extra fuel in the trunk, and it doesn't do you any good there!

TAKE NOTE

Geneen Roth popularized this concept of being hungry for something other than food in her groundbreaking book *When Food Is Love*, and has been a pioneer in the weight-loss field as an author and workshop leader for decades. Her latest groundbreaking book is called *Women Food and God*.

What are you so hungry for in your life? Many people have difficulty answering this question, so here are a few hints to prompt some self-reflection:

- Emotionally: Where in your life are you hungry emotionally?
- Physically: What are you really hungry for physically?
- Spiritually: What do you need in your life spiritually?

Emotional Hunger

Emotionally, we can feel hungry or empty when we feel depleted or we haven't been given enough of what we want in our lives—anything from love to time to attention. When we feel starved of love, starved for attention, or starved for enough time in our lives to give ourselves peace and stillness, we can reach out for a substitute such as extra food. While this makes perfect sense in the moment, it ends up hurting you.

Do you have enough love in your life? I don't mean romantic love; I mean, are you giving enough love to others, and are you receiving enough love from friends and family members who are grounded and centered enough to give you the time and space you deserve? Sometimes we are surrounded by people who are self-centered and lack the skills or maturity to listen and pay attention to us in a healthy, balanced, reciprocal relationship.

And of course, the most important source for love is from yourself. Are you giving yourself enough compassion, love, and respect? Or do you criticize yourself, break your own promises, and neglect your basic needs? We could all use more compassion and respect in our lives, and the first place to start is to give this to yourself. If you have been neglecting yourself by withholding love, compassion, or attention, you will certainly be hungry for something outside of yourself and might reach for food when the truth is you should be reaching for love.

TAPPING TIP

It's time to stop starving yourself of self-love. Take the time to write a quick list of what you appreciate about yourself—emotionally, as a friend, as an employee, as a family member—and consider how lucky those around you are to have you in their lives. Remember what's unique and special about you, and remind yourself often how you appreciate your gifts.

Physical Hunger

Consider your physical life and what's missing or what's out of balance. Is your body starving for exercise? Nature? Sunshine? Water? What are you missing in your life on a physical level that would trigger you to overeat even when you're not physically hungry?

Exercise has so many positive benefits for our bodies as well as for our minds, but it can be one of the first things to drop off of our to-do list when we're too busy. Or some of us never figured out how to put exercise into our lives to begin with. Exercise can dampen our appetite, raise our energy, and improve our mood, all of which are important for balance in our lives and to take the edge off an appetite that has been fueled by something that is missing. We're often trying to fill a void rather than actually feeling hungry for fuel for our bodies.

Spiritual Hunger

Spirituality is a profound part of our lives that we often neglect. I don't mean religion when I talk of spirituality. I mean connection to a power greater than yourself. I mean connecting to "source energy" or whatever you call life, energy, a deeper connection to the universe, or the divine. If none of those phrases appeal to you, you might consider nature to be something spiritual, or bigger than you, having a life and a cycle of its own.

A deep spiritual connection can form the fabric of a community and a family, so we ignore it at our peril. Are you spiritually hungry? Because if you're not plugged in to a spiritual dimension of your life, you might plug in to something else outside of yourself—food, drugs, alcohol, or drama, to name a few.

So again, ask the right questions:

- What are you truly hungry for?
- What are you seeking in your life?

I can promise you that food is not the answer—it never has been, although temporarily it can calm you down. And food is not successfully filling the void of what you feel you are missing in your life. That's why the cycle is so frustrating. We feel hungry; we reach for food; but the food doesn't truly satisfy us. It only makes us hungrier for what we truly need, and adds extra pounds to make us more upset and less satisfied in our lives!

▶ TAKING THE FIRST STEP

So before we identify the "real" problem with your weight-loss challenge, the first thing you need to do is give yourself some compassion for what you've been going through. You need to stop criticizing yourself for all the failures you catalogue about going up and down on the scale. You may have even been vulnerable enough to ask for help, yet not received the right help you needed. We know that 90 percent of restrictive diet plans don't work in the long term, and it's not your fault. You probably followed the food choices of your chosen new diet religiously for a long time, perplexed by why it wasn't working faster or for longer periods of time.

So it's time for you to appreciate all the efforts you have made, and recognize that you have not been given the right tools . . . until now. It's as if you have been trying to hammer a nail with a screwdriver. It's just not going to be that effective.

Remember the famous phrase: *Happiness is an inside job.* And so is successful weight loss. No outside substances, such as sugar, carbohydrates, or extra helpings of dessert, are going to make you happy or successful. You must learn how to tackle the uncomfortable feelings that make you feel scared or anxious, so you no longer need to reach out for extra food to calm you down. When you work on your inside—your feelings, emotional conflicts, and insecurities—your outside heals, too. It's worth the work.

▶ THE REAL WEIGHT-LOSS PROBLEM

Eating too much is the problem, right? You overeat three times a day and add several hundred calories in between meals. That's why your pants don't fit; that's why your suit is tight; and that's why you weigh more than you did last year when the doctor put you on the scale. That's the obvious answer. . . . Or is it?

Eating too much appears to be the cause of putting on the pounds and making your pants feel as if they've been through the wash and dry cycle too many times. But is eating too much actually the *real* problem? And if it is the real problem, why isn't it easier to stop overeating and lose weight?

Because eating too much isn't the problem; it's only a *symptom* of the problem.

This is good news, I promise. While you may feel discouraged that you've been targeting the wrong problem all of these years, and been wasting time struggling with all the diets you've tried in vain, wouldn't it be exciting to finally get to the bottom of your weight issue and overeating tendencies? And wouldn't it be relieving to finally reach and maintain your weight-loss goals? Remember: *it's not about the food!*

When I think of the time, calories, effort, and emotional bandwidth taken up with worrying about food, it's beyond frustrating. Part of why I'm so passionate about getting this information out to a wider audience is because I don't want people to suffer any more than they already have—seeing decades of misinformation, diet book seduction, and downright deceit in the diet industry is maddening. But you don't have to follow that path any longer. You can take a new journey, one that has a happy ending.

Now just because eating too much is only a symptom of the real problem, it doesn't mean you can continue to overeat and lose weight. It simply means that if you continue to focus on the food, you'll be chasing your tail and getting nowhere. I know 99 percent of you reading this book can relate to "getting nowhere" when it comes to your weight loss. It's depressing. It's discouraging. It's mind-boggling. Something doesn't add up. You wonder if you're defective, why dieting isn't working for you.

Before I discovered how to use tapping for weight loss, I just kept trying fad diets that never worked for more than a few months. I always lost the weight, but sadly, I always found it again. The results of these fad diets were predictably—and frustratingly—temporary.

So if eating too much isn't the real problem, then what is?

Learning to Manage Your Emotions

The real problem is that we don't know how (or never learned how) to manage our emotions, so we eat to cover up stress, anxiety, tension, hurt, anger, frustration, loneliness, and fear. If you don't know that a hammer is useful, you won't go looking for one—it's not in your toolbox yet. I've recently introduced you to the right tool, though: *tapping*.

What gets you stuck in any area of your life are your fears, feelings, and beliefs. But somehow, even when you've asked for help, you haven't been led to the right tools to clear these fears, feelings, and beliefs. Typically, not enough attention is paid to these emotions and conflicts, or to the emotional risks of losing weight. Whether these perceived risks are conscious or unconscious doesn't matter; they aren't given enough attention and treatment for success to take hold.

You have dozens of emotions every day, and have had millions of feelings course through your body and mind throughout your lifetime. That doesn't mean you're good at recognizing or managing them. It just means they are a part of life, and it's a good idea to learn how to handle them so you don't resort to food, alcohol, cigarettes, sex, or drama to obliterate them.

--- **TAPPING TIP** ---

Pause and write down as many emotions as you've felt today and connect them to a point in time in your life. For instance, "I felt worried when my boss gave me an extra assignment due next week" or "I felt lonely on Friday night when I didn't have any plans with friends." Notice how many you have in just one hour!

When you think about it, eating more food than is served in a regular meal is kind of strange, isn't it? If you eat when you're physically hungry, you should be able to stop when you're full and satisfied. This sounds logical enough, and is logical to people who never learned how to use food to tranquilize their emotions.

But when you're eating for reasons other than hunger, you don't stop; you can't stop, because something more important takes over: the need to emotionally survive.

Having too many strong emotions that you don't know what to do with causes you to disconnect from the actual physical hunger that signals you when you're biologically hungry, and you start eating for other, more emotional reasons. It becomes more important to your brain and actually to your survival to numb your feelings than to stick to a diet. This is why, in spite of your claims that "this time I'm really sticking to it," you fall off the wagon yet again. When your feelings are too strong or painful, they take over and rule your behavior. And if you don't have a tool to manage your feelings, you are a sitting duck for resorting to unhealthy behaviors such as overeating.

The Limits of Logical Thinking

When stress, worry, or fear is driving you to overeat, then stopping eating isn't logical and it won't make sense. For starters, when you're in the middle of trying desperately to calm down your emotions, you're not thinking logically. And secondly, when your first priority is to calm your feelings, it doesn't matter whether your behavior makes sense or not; you don't care anymore. This is how, day after day and eventually year after year, you gain weight, stretch your stomach, and come to ignore natural signals of hunger and satiety.

Why? Because the need to shut down your worry or quiet your stress is even more important than biology, and in fact, it can even override your biological signals that are trying to get your attention.

Human beings want to survive. It's a biological imperative. So when something threatens our survival, we'll move heaven and earth to find safety. Now think about feeling unsafe, worried, or frustrated. It feels scary, sometimes overwhelming, hinting at a threat to your survival. So instead of listening to the biology that says, "I'm full, I don't need a third helping at dinner," your mind and body say: "I can't afford to feel this worry; I think another helping will shut it up the way it did the last time, and the time before that."

So while overeating evidently puts on the pounds, trying to anesthetize your emotions is the *real* reason you are overeating. If you change food plans, the success can only be temporary. If you address the real cause of being overweight—overeating because you don't want to feel certain emotions—the results can be permanent and satisfying.

▶ THE MISSING LINK

Learning to understand your emotional triggers and calming them down is what has been missing for decades in the toolbox offered by the diet industry—not the perfect combination of food choices, or a different list of what to eat, or a calendar of when to eat it, but a tool to manage the triggers that cause us to reach for extra food. A tool to calm us down naturally, in a healthy, quick way, so we can face the challenges that life throws our way. That tool, as you learned in Chapter 1, is called tapping.

I didn't know about tapping until eighteen years ago. But I use the tool in my current life to handle daily feelings of stress, worry, and anxiety, and I can also use it on conflicts from decades ago—feelings and memories that can heap on more stress and make me want to overeat.

Yes, tapping is just a tool, but it's the best tool I have discovered in over twenty years in the mental health field. And tapping can be used for every step of your weight-loss journey. It is versatile and simple, and you can use it on yourself as many times a day as you need it.

▶ THE PROBLEM IS THE SOLUTION

Let's start with the premise that changed my life and my work: If there is a big problem in your life, this problem was once a solution; it has just gotten out of control for you. In other words, maybe you procrastinated to avoid being criticized. Did it work? Yes, temporarily. But then of course it caused new problems—your boss is mad because your work is never on time. But at least you didn't fail, because you never got the work done so you could never get evaluated! This may sound backwards, but it's how our minds work. We all want to be protected, and if our mind makes us procrastinate because it gets us out of a jam, or prevents us from being judged, that behavior will win the day.

The attitude that the challenge you hate so much about yourself is actually an attempt to solve a problem is very useful for a couple of reasons. First of all, it's the truth! You wouldn't behave in a way that appears to sabotage your deepest dreams if it wasn't accomplishing a positive result for you on some level. Second of all, once you understand this motivation behind the problem—once you identify the problem it was trying to solve—you can address the real problem and clear it for good.

Until you identify what you were trying to solve with your negative behavior, you can never enjoy permanent success. Think about it. Wouldn't it be awesome if you could finally get to the bottom of why you keep sabotaging yourself? You'll need to stop criticizing yourself for this behavior of sabotage or else the real work can never begin.

The same theory goes for people with the fear of success or the fear of failure. It works for people who smoke, people who procrastinate, and for people who date inappropriate and unavailable partners in spite of claiming "I want to be married."

So from now on, whenever you encounter a behavior in yourself or others that looks crazy, destructive, stupid, or sabotaging, consider this:

- What does the behavior do that is positive?
- What does it provide that is comforting?
- How does it make me (or the other person) feel better in the moment?

When you're aware that taking away the behavior is threatening, you'll better understand why it is such a struggle to put down the cigarettes, the drink, the bag of chips, or the partner who thrives on drama.

▶ FIND YOUR WHY

So let's start with this all-important question: *Do you know why you yo-yo?*

If you have gone up and down on the scale more than once, it's important to identify why you can't keep the weight off. What if there's a good reason for you to yo-yo that's not physiological or biological? What if your mind is creating part of this puzzle? What if you are actually trying to protect yourself emotionally or physically with the extra weight, so that any attempts to lose the weight will automatically backfire?

Chances are you never considered that there may be psychological advantages to keeping the weight on. You may consciously know about them ("I feel safer with extra weight"), but you probably never incorporated this information into your food plan or exercise regimen. And as a result, yo-yoing has probably been inevitable, every time.

Does this sound familiar?

You're inspired to lose weight; you found a new food plan that you think you can stick with; you eat healthier meals, smaller portions, and even start a walking program. The scale is your friend. You start to see progress in your weight as the number on the scale goes down. You're doing fine, sailing along, when bam! You hit a wall. You start thinking about sweets; you start cheating on your food plan; you hear yourself saying, "I'll get back on my diet tomorrow." Tomorrow turns into a long string of days, and the needle on the scale starts going in the wrong direction.

What happened? Where did that motivated "I can do it" person go? Why are the sweets beyond tempting again? Why are those fattening foods calling your name every five minutes? Are you crazy or just out of control? Are you indifferent, or is this blatant sabotage of your progress?

I'm here to tell you that you are not crazy. In fact, you are incredibly logical and smart, and are attempting to keep yourself safe and content. Only the way you've chosen to do it has negative side effects and is making you unhappy. But if you measure which is more important to you—being overweight versus feeling safe in your body and your environment—being safe will win every time. That's why the food wins every time; you haven't tackled the safety issue.

CASE STUDY

Susan felt inspired to finally lose the extra twenty-five pounds that had been creeping up over the years. She felt uncomfortable in her body, didn't have enough energy for her kids, and didn't like the way she looked. She felt it was finally time to focus on her weight-loss goal and do the work she needed to do.

She dropped her extra weight quickly, and was happy with herself. Her clothes fit; she had more energy; and the compliments were plentiful. She said that it seemed so easy this time. But after a few days at her new goal weight, she found herself eating uncontrollably and was utterly baffled by her behavior. She said it felt as if there was someone inside of her compulsively chasing food, as if she wasn't connected to this behavior. It might have seemed illogical, but it wasn't. It turned out that being overweight was a safety issue for Susan.

I asked her if being at the lower weight scared her in any way, and she had to admit that she felt more vulnerable and visible without her extra protection. Susan recounted a frightening story of when she had been sexually attacked as a teenager, and admitted that the extra weight served as some kind of armor for her. She knew it didn't sound rational, but it felt better to have extra protection on her. After tapping on this fear of being attacked, and understanding the origin of the fear was the incident that had so threatened her, she was able to get her eating back under control and feel safe losing the weight again.

Everyone who has sabotaged their progress on a weight-loss plan has been deeply disappointed and discouraged by their behavior. They usually get mad at themselves and criticize their sabotage behavior. The problem with this reaction is that it leaves no room for psychological exploration about why they would feel the urge to sabotage. If all that noise from the criticism and judgment is taking up space in your mind, how could you come up with positive solutions or insights that could be the game-changer that you've been looking for all these years?

So why would you sabotage your progress? What's in it for you? How does it help you? Remember that each problem we have was once a solution. It served a purpose for us, even though it has now become a problem.

Here are my two favorite questions to use in my coaching program and psychotherapy practice:

1. What's the *upside* to holding on to this problem?
2. What's the *downside* to getting over it?

Early on, overeating was probably incredibly effective for calming down your feelings, but now, later in life, you have put the pounds on; you hate your body; and you can't get your eating habits or your weight back under control. So finding your "why" is essential here. Why is it so important to have extra weight on you, or why is it so helpful to eat so much outside of meals and even when you're not hungry?

CASE STUDY

Mary worked for a year to lose more than one hundred pounds. She posted photographs on the Internet; she wrote blogs about her success; she gave advice to friends and family. However, the reaction to her success wasn't all positive. After she had lost all the weight she had struggled with over the years, her family didn't appear to be very happy about it. In fact, they seemed downright hostile to her.

Instead of getting approval and compliments from her family members, she weathered their irritation, frustration, and criticism. They said she seemed "too serious" and no fun anymore. They accused her of being judgmental of their weight problems. Mary started eating compulsively, secretly, and regularly, and sure enough the pounds started to come back on.

Fortunately, Mary recognized what was happening and thought about why she was responding in this way. After much thought and consideration, she came up with two conclusions. First, her family members were too jealous to be able to handle her success, and second, now she felt as if she didn't belong in this family anymore. Even though she had wanted emotional freedom from them for years, and recognized their toxic communication habits, now that she didn't belong she wanted to be a part of the group again. The upside to staying fat would be to fit in her family; the downside of losing the weight was that she didn't belong anymore. Once Mary recognized this, she was able to effectively use tapping on her fears, her panic, and her compulsive behavior. She was able to stabilize her behavior and her weight.

▶ FEAR OF FAILURE AND FEAR OF SUCCESS

I coach many people on how to eliminate procrastination and sabotage behavior, and nine times out of ten, the reason they sabotage is because of their fear of failure or their fear of success. What's the difference? One group fears that their efforts will end in failure and humiliation, and the other group fears that people will envy and resent them because of their success.

So when you procrastinate your weight-loss plan, ask yourself: *What are you afraid of?* Sometimes you feel so burned by your past attempts at weight loss that you don't want to risk it again. Other times you're not quite sure why you sabotaged your plan last time, so you don't think it's smart to try again . . . so you keep putting it off. Many of my clients have said to me, "If I lose the weight and I'm still not happy, then what?"

Exactly. Would that read as a failure to you? If you lose the weight and are still unhappy, does that mean you don't know the answer to making you happy? What happens to all the time and effort you put into hating yourself for being overweight? What if it's not the issue at all?

These are huge challenges for people, and they need to be addressed emotionally and psychologically, not with calorie counting. See if you can figure out any other failures you might be afraid of if you are *successful* at losing the weight.

And if you are totally successful and happy this time, and find the keys to losing and keeping the weight off, and stop using food to manage your emotions, what's the risk? Why are you afraid of success? Usually the answers center around other people's reactions. Some possible fears could be:

- "My friends/family/others won't like me anymore."
- "They won't like it that I've lost weight and they haven't."
- "They will give me a hard time for focusing on my appearance."
- "They will be jealous of my success."

CASE STUDY

One client, Allison, didn't want to take the heat from her sister, who also had a weight problem. She knew that not only would her sister tempt her to overeat when they were together; she would likely be mean about the whole issue because she had never been able to lose the weight herself. Adding even more conflict in her family, her mother gave her food every time she walked in the door! She definitely didn't know how to handle this behavior, so it was easier for her to stay the same.

Allison wasn't sure what to do with the conflict she had and the feeling that staying the same was easier than making changes. I helped her tap for her fear of her sister's reaction, and the temptation when her mother gave her extra food. She immediately felt more confident and less afraid of their reactions. She started to understand their emotional discomfort with her progress, and decided it was not her job to make them feel better. We tapped on her guilt about her success, her fear that she was being disloyal by being the only family member successful at weight loss, and her ongoing cravings that surfaced when she was under stress. She tapped every day on her cravings, and even though they felt physical and real to her—that she had to eat something right away—she soon realized that her cravings were always stress-related.

After she had lost twenty-one pounds, she went to visit her mother, and sure enough, her mother gave her a frozen chocolate pie as a "gift" when she was leaving. Allison had no interest in eating it, had compassion for what her mother must have been feeling when she gave her the pie ("she wouldn't take no for an answer"), and felt calm and peaceful on her drive home. She was amazed at how much tapping had helped her with losing weight, but appreciated her new self-confidence as well. She appreciated being less entangled emotionally with her family, yet she still loved them, visited them, and honored their feelings.

To avoid social or familial discomfort, we often sabotage our success. It's easier; it keeps things in balance; it doesn't rock the boat. However, it can make you miserable. Other people's reactions to your success aren't your problems to fix. So how about doing this for you, not for them, regardless of their reactions?

Think of any other reasons you might be afraid of success. Are you afraid of getting unwanted attention from others? Romantic attention? Someone might notice you more? When these two key reasons to sabotage—fear of failure and fear of success—are addressed and healed with tapping, then your mind and body won't support the sabotage behavior anymore. There's no need to. Sabotage ceases to become urgent or life-saving for your mind and body, so you don't do it anymore.

▶ SAFETY AND IDENTITY ISSUES

There are two primary areas of sabotage that don't get enough attention: safety and identity. Remember that you absolutely—biologically and emotionally—need to feel safe. You need to feel safe in your environment, in your body, in your home, and in your relationships. And when you don't feel safe, you will do anything that is within your power to become safer, even if those behaviors look bizarre to the outside world.

If you don't feel safe in your work environment because the boss is always yelling at you and your coworkers seem ready to throw you under the bus, the chronic anxiety of spending forty to sixty hours a week in this environment might make you feel threatened, even though nothing physically dangerous would ever happen there. As a result, you might resort to overeating just to calm your nerves, to block out the noise of all the agitation that goes on day in and day out, to make you feel emotionally safe by being bigger and taking up more space.

If you don't feel comfortable in your own body, in your own skin, you will also behave in a way that covers you up and hides who you are.

CASE STUDY

A client of mine, Sarah, always felt criticized by her brothers and her father. They ridiculed her, laughed at her, and said she wasn't smart. She learned to use food as comfort at an early age, since she never felt safe when speaking her mind. When she got her first adult job, she felt the same lack of safety with her boss and coworkers, and an adolescent eating disorder returned until she got control of her emotions and her deep feeling of being threatened.

Sarah contacted me for tapping for what she called her "social anxiety." She never felt comfortable speaking up at work or at work functions, and she continued to feel "less than" in front of her father and brothers. Her food cravings had subsided with some of the tapping she did on herself; however, she would occasionally binge eat before or after one of these upsetting and anxiety-provoking work events.

We tapped on her fear of being ridiculed, the memories of her family members actually teasing her, and her fear of speaking up in a crowd. She needed to do significant tapping on some of the old memories of events when her father was particularly cruel and taunting. Her anxiety decreased dramatically, and even more exciting for her, her binge eating stopped!

We continued to tap on her relationship with her boss as a scary authority figure and continued to tap on her self-worth until she started to agree that yes, she was valuable and that she had something valuable to say! She continued to tap on her own on a daily basis; her weight totally stabilized; and her social anxiety continued to decrease.

Now let's talk about identity issues. If you have been struggling with your weight, with diets, and with body shame for a few years or a few decades, consider this question: Who are you going to be when you reach your goal weight?

How are you going to feel about yourself when you no longer have this problem to worry about? When I asked a client why she was sabotaging her eating plan, she said, "Who on earth am I going to be without this problem? It's been my identity for thirty years. I don't want to lose it." This both made perfect sense and seemed utterly insane to her at the same time! It was imperative that she uncovered this mode of sabotage so she could release the attachment to her problem and move forward.

So if you suspect you have safety or identity issues regarding your weight, your body, and your place in the world, stay tuned for some sample tapping sequences that will soothe your heart and soul so you no longer have to hide from everyone, including yourself.

▶ EXPLORE THE DOWNSIDE

Remember that the first key question to get to the bottom of your cycling up and down on the scale is deceptively simple: What is the downside to losing the weight?

For some people, this question stops them in their tracks. For others, they know exactly what the answer is. Were you able to answer this question? *What is the downside to losing the weight?*

Other ways of asking this question, which might help you get to the clues and core answers about why you won't give up all the extra food, are: *What are you afraid of if you lose the weight? What is something negative that might come out of losing the weight?*

I'm going to give you some examples of answers my clients have given me over the years. Please put a check mark next to any of these sample answers that are true for you:

❑ If I lose the weight, I don't trust myself to keep it off.
❑ If I lose the weight, I don't know if I can maintain my goal.
❑ If I lose the weight, I'll get way too much attention from others.
❑ If I lose the weight, I'll get unwanted romantic attention.
❑ If I lose the weight, someone will be jealous and mean to me.
❑ I'm afraid of the anger that might surface when I'm not eating.
❑ I'm afraid of all my emotions that might show up if I lose the weight.
❑ What if I start remembering those traumas again?
❑ What if there are buried memories I'm avoiding?
❑ If I lose the weight, I won't feel like I belong in my family.
❑ Who will I be if I'm no longer the heavy one in my family?
❑ Who will I be if I'm no longer the friend with the weight problem?
❑ If I lose the weight, I won't recognize myself.
❑ I've been this way so long, it won't feel normal to lose the weight.
❑ If I lose the weight, someone will accuse me of being self-centered.
❑ If I lose the weight, my spouse/partner will sabotage me.
❑ If I lose the weight, I have to get a whole new set of clothes.
❑ If I lose the weight, I won't have a project to work on.
❑ If I lose the weight, I might still be unhappy. Then what?
❑ If I lose the weight, I'll feel deprived.
❑ If I lose the weight, something bad might happen to me.

- ❏ If I lose the weight, I won't feel safe.
- ❏ If I lose the weight, I'll feel exposed or vulnerable.
- ❏ If I lose the weight, they won't notice me anymore.
- ❏ If I lose the weight, I'm more vulnerable to attack.

Get the picture? There are lots of reasons you might feel afraid or have mixed feelings about losing weight, but *none of these reasons can be addressed by fancy fad diet strategies*. That's why you haven't been successful yet (and yes, I mean *yet*).

▶ EXPLORE THE UPSIDE

Now for our next question under the "why do you yo-yo" topic: *What's the upside to staying overweight?* Again, here are some answers that my clients have given me over the years. Do any of them resonate with you?

- ❏ If I stay overweight, I don't have to do that much work.
- ❏ If I stay overweight, I don't have to worry about my meals.
- ❏ If I stay overweight, I don't have to plan around social events.
- ❏ If I stay overweight, I don't have to do anything about my clothes.
- ❏ When I'm overweight, I feel protected by my weight.
- ❏ When I'm overweight, I don't have to put up with extra attention.
- ❏ If I stay overweight, I don't have to feel deprived.
- ❏ If I stay overweight, I can just relax around my sugar issues.
- ❏ If I stay overweight, I don't have to waste any more time dieting.
- ❏ If I stay overweight, I don't have to feel ashamed when I regain it.
- ❏ When I'm overweight, no one has any expectations of me.
- ❏ If I stay overweight, I don't have to do more in my life.
- ❏ If I stay overweight, I can take the pressure off of me to diet.

❑ When I'm overweight, I won't feel pressured to improve.

❑ If I stay overweight, I can just stop worrying about this problem.

❑ If I stay overweight, I can just keep eating when I want to.

❑ If I stay overweight, I can give up the dream of being thin one day.

❑ If I stay overweight, I can enjoy food again.

❑ If I stay overweight, I can continue to keep people away from me.

❑ If I stay overweight, I don't have to enter an intimate relationship.

❑ If I stay overweight, I can just be me and stop worrying about this.

There are many more answers that might occur to you about the *upside* of staying overweight. Feel free to add to this list—anything that seems like a plus to staying the way you are. Another way of asking my question would be to ask, "How does this problem serve you?" Look around your life and see how this problem helps you out physically, mentally, emotionally, or socially.

These fears—of being exposed, scrutinized, or vulnerable—are the real reasons you keep yo-yoing up and down the scale.

Remember: if it feels better to be safe with anywhere from twenty to one hundred extra pounds on your frame, you will move heaven and earth to make this happen. If you feel stronger because you feel bigger, you'll stay bigger, regardless of calorie counting. If you think being visible is unsafe, and being big makes you somehow invisible to others, you will do anything it takes to remain big in your eyes.

We're dealing with perception here: perception of safety, perception of value, perception of what makes sense. Your friend may not think it makes sense that you are carrying an extra fifty pounds on you to be invisible, but if your subconscious mind thinks it's a good idea, you will absolutely do what it takes to carry that extra weight. Safety is the name of the game—physically, emotionally, and mentally.

So let's continue to address the culprits that cause us to sabotage our behavior—the real reasons you are overweight.

▶ STRESS AND WEIGHT GAIN

What's too often missing from the discussion of obesity in our society is the role that stress plays in this societal and physical challenge.

Stress can cause us to sabotage our weight-loss plan because we feel depleted and exhausted, and stress hormones start to interfere with our mood and biology. Cortisol, a hormone released when you're in danger, starts coursing through your body, and it can actually cause you to hold more weight around your midsection.

Stress is our *perception* of external demands on us. Ten of us could have the exact same situation at work with the same boss, but we each would respond differently to it—we would respond with different emotions, which means our bodies would also respond differently. So it's important to remember that what *you* consider stressful may not stress out your neighbor. The point is we are all overwhelmed with stressful situations—some acute, some chronic—and how we handle what happens in our life determines our emotional and physical health and strength.

TAKE NOTE

Hans Selye, a Hungarian-born researcher and scientist, is considered the "father" of the stress movement. He was the first to coin the term "the Stress Response," which he accidentally stumbled upon during research for another project. Selye considered stress our reaction to any outside circumstances that feel like a demand to us. He authored numerous books and scientific papers, the most famous of which is *The Stress of Life*. He also was a pioneer in making the connection between long-term stress and physical illnesses.

Sadly, some of us are totally unaware of what is causing us to feel stressed in our daily lives. Sometimes we are so overwhelmed that all we can do is just get by. For example, maybe we feel good because at least we fed the dog today. Stress affects our sleep, our eating, our relationships, and our social life.

What events or situations in your day or week cause you the most stress? Family conflict? Work deadlines? Your health? Being on another diet? How about getting on the scale? I have a client who feels so stressed out about needing to weigh herself that the stress causes her to overeat!

Ironically, the restrictive nature of a diet triggers stress hormones in our bodies, too—working against us right when we most want to be losing weight. The stress response triggers a cascade of chemicals in our bodies that are terrible for us, cause us to hold on to weight, or make it harder to let excess weight go. So if you haven't been focused on reducing the stress in your life, you are barking up the wrong tree.

If we feel hurt, angry, frustrated, or resentful, it triggers a stress response inside of us, because of our perception of the environment's demands on us, and starts this negative process in our bodies. You might feel powerless on the job, or aggravated with your teenagers, or exasperated by a traffic jam when you're late for an appointment. How do you handle this? Does it feel like a crisis? Does it feel as if you can take it in stride? Do you feel overheated emotionally when something seemingly small occurs in your day? So many small things can trigger our stress response. We don't even see our stress response coming, and we certainly don't know how to stop it in the middle of our reaction.

Sadly, when we have a great deal of stress in our lives, we become less resilient to new or ongoing demands. So if work is particularly challenging this month, or the kids are all sick with the flu this week, you end up being less competent at handling stress in a calm way. Basically, your resources get used up, and if you're not recharging your battery every day, then you eventually feel emotionally and physically depleted, and unable to handle what's showing up in your emotional inbox.

As I discussed earlier, we overeat because we want to anesthetize our uncomfortable or upsetting emotions. So being on the right food plan doesn't change this unless you are supported by the right tools to handle your emotions. There's nothing wrong with a sensible food plan, unless you don't have a way to embrace and release your strong emotions.

Our response to stress becomes an automatic reaction, and if you don't use tools to take care of this reactivity and reduce your heated responses, you will naturally move toward using food to calm you down.

Remember: food works to calm you. It's hard to be frustrated when you're focused on a pint of ice cream or a bag of chips. That's the point: Food is being used for a "good" reason—at least your brain thinks it's a good idea in the moment. The fact that using extra food makes you fall off your healthy eating program, gain weight, and feel ashamed or unhappy with yourself is irrelevant at the time! You have one goal in mind when the stress overwhelms you—one purpose, and that's to eliminate your negative feelings as quickly as possible.

So until you get your stress under control, it's unlikely that you will get your overeating under control. They work together to sabotage your success every time.

TAPPING TIP

Take the time to write a list of other ways you could reward yourself besides food. Remember: food works to soothe your feelings in the moment, but what else would work? A fresh glass of water, a slow, peaceful walk, calming music, or a talk with a friend? Enjoy writing the list and then enjoy feeling better after indulging in these healthy rewards!

▶ BODY IMAGE

Do you like your body? Have you ever liked your body? When you look in the mirror, do you ever say anything nice about what you see? I bet all of you reading this book answered "no" to at least one of the previous questions.

Imagine all the stress it creates when you have this constant mind chatter that says, "I'm so fat" or "I look terrible" or "I hate my thighs." Remember the cascade of stress hormones we talked about, and how they can actually signal your body to hold on to weight? This is what you're releasing into your bloodstream when you constantly criticize your body.

What I know for certain is that you wouldn't talk to a friend of yours this way, because you know it wouldn't do any good, and in fact, you know that it might even make things worse! Yet you find it acceptable to talk to yourself this way.

What if you stopped beating up your body? What if you started appreciating your body and its strengths and stopped looking for the perfect shape as displayed in Madison Avenue magazines? What if you could enjoy a deep sense of relaxation from releasing all this negativity? It would definitely be healthier for your body and mind.

I want you to start being an ally to your body rather than its enemy. It's always easier to get a project done when all the people (or parts) involved are working in harmony, in unison. When all of you is rooting for success, appreciating what's good, and wanting the same thing, you will be more likely to achieve your goal.

In addition to the fact that this constant barrage of negative talk triggers stress hormones to run through your body, it also doesn't help you lose weight. In fact, it can slow down your progress, in spite of what you're eating. I know, we were taught that we would become more motivated if we were disgusted with ourselves and wanted to change. The truth is, negativity slows us down—and it attracts the weight to us because we are so invested in hating it.

Do you know the difference between motivation and inspiration? Motivation only lasts a few days or a few weeks, while inspiration can last a lifetime. Think of it this way: When all those eager gym enthusiasts start out their New Year's resolutions by trying new workouts in the gym, the ones who quit in February were using motivation. The ones who are still there in the spring felt inspired to take care of themselves, and they are sticking with it because it feels good, not because it's a punishment. These people who were inspired truly desire a healthier body and a healthier lifestyle. They're not making themselves walk because they've had a bad week or month.

Self-acceptance is a key piece to the tapping method I described in Chapter 1, and one that you will learn to use to relieve your uncomfortable emotions. In fact, during each round of the tapping sequences, you will be saying a statement of acceptance about the problem you have chosen to work on. What's the point? When you finally accept your feelings or your conflicts, this creates psychological space for change, for creativity, for resourcefulness and inspiration. Accepting your feelings and your situation reduces the self-inflicted pressure, which will allow you to move forward instead of staying stuck.

So if you want your weight-loss journey to be easier, try being easier on your body. Try appreciating parts of your body that have helped you, that have shown strength and longevity. Try noticing what looks good. The result? You'll feel better, which will help you feel more inspired, which will help you make healthier food choices starting today!

Think about it. If you hated your dinner guests, would you go to any trouble to make them a nice, healthy meal? No! You wouldn't care what you fed them!

It's also a good idea to consider where you learned how to talk this way. The self-talk may be so automatic, you don't know where it originally came from or why you keep doing it. Maybe you learned it from an older sister, or your mother or father. Maybe you saw other women talking this way. Once you become more conscious of where it came from or where you learned it, you will be able to recognize it when it starts and stop it midsentence. Yes, you can learn to stop it and then replace it with new language, new self-talk, and new patterns of behavior that are working for you, not against you.

Before reading any further, see if you can make a list of what you appreciate about your body—any parts, any functions, your best features, its strengths. Work on this every day and you will wonder why you haven't been doing this exercise all along.

CHAPTER SUMMARY

In this chapter:

- We discussed why diets don't work—because they make you feel deprived, signal your metabolism to slow down, and don't target the real reason you're overweight.

- We looked at the real reason why you're overeating and its connection to emotional and spiritual voids you may have in your life.

- We learned how the inability to handle our uncomfortable feelings leads to eating instead of healing the hurt.

- We explored the reasons people sabotage themselves when they try to lose weight, including fear of success and fear of failure.

- We looked at the connection between safety and identity issues and your struggle to lose weight.

- We saw how stress creates a situation where it is extremely difficult to lose weight.

- We discovered how body image, particularly hating your body, plays a role in having difficulty losing weight, and how learning to appreciate your body can change this.

CHAPTER 3

TAPPING FOR WEIGHT LOSS

There is so much good news about using tapping for weight loss! In this chapter, we'll explore more specifically how to use tapping to help you address the emotional issues and responses that make it difficult for you to lose weight. We'll look at a variety of tapping exercises that you can use to help you meet your weight-loss goals, with each exercise targeting a different type of emotional or stress response. You'll be guided through the steps to take whether you're struggling with fear, anxiety, anger, or other emotions.

We'll also explore the many different ways you can create your setup statements in order to address the fears and emotional responses that are holding you back from losing weight. Creating an affirmative setup statement is one of the most crucial parts of the tapping process.

In addition, you'll learn a number of different tapping scripts to experiment with, as some will resonate more with you than others. (You'll find additional tapping scripts in Chapter 5.)

▶ WHEN TO USE TAPPING FOR WEIGHT LOSS

I know you have felt discouraged dozens of times on your weight-loss journey, but now there are many reasons for hope. You can use the technique of tapping to address every angle of your weight-loss challenge: cravings, plateaus, frustration, and stress relief. This versatility is why tapping is so effective. While I know you've been offered the latest fad diets, pills, and exercise programs, you've never been offered a tool this efficient and comprehensive before. So when should you use tapping for weight loss? Read on!

Immediate Cravings

You can use tapping when you have immediate cravings. When you feel the urge to eat something sweet or fatty to calm you down, this is an excellent time to use tapping, but it is often challenging to do it at the right time. The cravings can sometimes be so overwhelming, people who know how to tap actually forget to use this tool and reach for food instead.

This is why I invite people to schedule tapping into their day at least once or twice to handle the basic stress in their life from their job, family, or health concerns. This will help reduce the overall feelings of stress and being out of control. Reducing this overall stress will, over time, also reduce the number of times you get hit with those signals of cravings that seem truly irresistible. Release the stress, and you will release the cravings.

Deprivation

Do you feel deprived when you start a new diet? Does it always feel as if something is being taken away from you, or do you feel deprived of something that you need and want? Many people struggle on diets because dieting sets them up to feel emotionally deprived. And when they feel deprived, they feel compelled to rebel against the controls, and they start overeating to prove they are in charge.

TAPPING TIP

If suffering with feelings of deprivation is a challenge for you, rest assured that tapping is an excellent tool to help release your current feelings of deprivation, as well as feelings of deprivation from your past. Maybe you felt deprived of love, deprived of attention, or deprived of appreciation. When you tap to release these memories you will notice how your feelings subside and your cravings go away.

Frustration

You can use tapping on your frustration when the scale isn't responding fast enough for you. We are all way too attached to the number on the scale, myself included. Somehow we think a number is magic; when we get there, we'll be fine; and if we don't arrive at the magic number, our day is ruined. This is an awful way to live, and tapping is an excellent tool to handle the disappointment over what the scale says, as well as to handle the attachment you have developed to the number on the scale.

Plateaus

You can also use tapping when you hit the classic plateaus that you inevitably face each and every time you try and lose weight. Have you ever known anyone who didn't hit that wall at some point during a weight-loss program? Probably not. A plateau is when your body seems stuck at a certain weight on the journey down. It doesn't seem to budge regardless of what you're eating, and it can be exasperating. You feel frustrated, aggravated, and tempted to throw in the towel: "It's not working anyway. Why bother? What's the use?" All of these feelings and frustrations can be addressed with tapping.

Social Fear and Anxiety

What about when your fears and anxiety surface when you need to attend a work function or a social gathering, and all those tempting foods are staring you in the face? What then? This is an extremely challenging time for people who have started out on a healthy food plan. Their intentions are to stick to it, but combining the anxiety about being with work colleagues with being around free food can trigger the urge to overeat. Luckily, you can learn how to use tapping for the anxiety and the cravings, before, during, and after the social gathering!

Relapsing

I'm not perfect and don't pretend to want to be anymore. And you won't be perfect either, so remember: You can use tapping when you feel guilty for falling off your healthy food plan. This will help you stop the slide into relapse when you're feeling guilty or discouraged that you blew it again. Target the feelings of guilt and regret about going off your healthy diet, and tap on the discouragement about your behavior.

Confidence

You can use tapping for gaining confidence in your life and focusing more on your strengths and less on the number on the scale. You can target the reasons you have low self-esteem and release those feelings, fears, and assumptions that have been limiting you for so long. You may be overweight, but you're not a bad person. You may have yo-yoed up and down a few times, but you have value and worth and heart. Don't let this problem get the best of you. It's not worth it.

Emotions and Stress

You don't need more food for body fuel, you overeat because of stress and emotions that are swirling around in your life with no release. Tapping on fear, guilt, loneliness, stress, anger, resentment, and hurt will change your life on so many levels. Using the tool of tapping on all these emotions will reduce your overall stress levels, which will allow you to drop some of the extra weight you've been holding on to for safety reasons.

▶ *THE TAPPING DIET* METHOD

I recommend to clients that they tap at least twice a day, but remember that you can tap whenever you feel stressed, feel overwhelmed, or are tempted to eat even when you aren't truly hungry. In Chapter 4, we'll talk specifically about how to incorporate tapping into your daily life by making an action plan. For now, realize that daily attention to tapping will help you succeed in overcoming your weight-loss challenges.

As described in Chapter 2, there are five crucial steps involved in *The Tapping Diet* method:

1. Define a target (an emotion, a symptom, a belief, or a memory of an event)
2. Measure your level of distress
3. Create and use a setup statement
4. Tap on specific acupuncture points
5. Measure your level of distress again

Let's look more closely at each of these in turn.

The Tapping Diet Method: Step 1

The first step in the tapping method is to define a target for tapping. These targets can be:

- Emotions
- Memories of past experiences
- Negative or limiting beliefs
- Physical symptoms

Let's look at how each of these targets might connect with weight loss.

TAPPING TARGET: EMOTIONS

The best target for tapping is one of your emotions. Worry and stress are common triggers for overeaters. Here are some possible emotional situations that could be sabotaging your weight-loss efforts:

❑ My performance review at work is coming up and I'm concerned about how I'll do.

❑ I'm concerned that this physical pain is a sign of a bigger medical issue.

❑ I'm afraid there won't be enough money for a vacation again this year.

❑ I'm so stressed-out about the school conferences for the kids this year.

❑ I'm worried about the changes going on at work, and whether they will still need me.

❑ I feel intense stress about the holidays coming up.

❑ I feel insecure about going to this work event. What if I don't measure up?

❑ I feel worried and anxious that I'm not going to fit in when we all get together this weekend.

❑ I feel frustrated and irritable because I'm not getting enough sleep these days.

❑ I feel worried about all my deadlines at work right now.

❑ I feel hurt by what my friend said to me, and I don't know how to deal with it.

❑ I feel lonely a lot these days, and I don't feel comfortable reaching out to people.

❑ I feel angry about being underappreciated at work, but I don't know how to talk to my boss.

❑ I feel resentful that I'm not getting enough support at home.

❑ I feel scared of making the upcoming changes in my life. How will I handle it all?

TAPPING TARGET: MEMORIES OF PAST EXPERIENCES

If you're planning to tap to deal with a memory of a past event, it may be beneficial and advisable to seek additional professional help. If memories are deeply upsetting from your past, you may automatically avoid working on them to protect yourself from the emotional pain. So you will never be able to get to the bottom of the problem because you don't feel safe *going there*.

However, if you feel safe working on a past memory, you may be able to find that a past event ties in to your weight-loss difficulties. Perhaps you experienced scarcity and lack, or didn't get what you wanted. The memory of that event could be sabotaging your present-day efforts at weight loss. Here are some great examples of past experiences that may have taught you to console yourself with food:

- ❏ The time I failed the test and the teacher yelled at me.
- ❏ The time the coach humiliated me in front of my classmates.
- ❏ The time my father hit me.
- ❏ The time my grandmother died and no one listened to me.
- ❏ The time the teacher said I would never amount to anything.
- ❏ The time I fell and broke my wrist.
- ❏ The time I was left out when they chose sides for the soccer team.
- ❏ The time I was physically abused.
- ❏ The time I was sexually abused.
- ❏ The time I was neglected.
- ❏ The time they said [fill in the blank].
- ❏ The time they did [fill in the blank].
- ❏ The time I didn't feel safe because [fill in the blank].

TAPPING TARGET: NEGATIVE OR LIMITING BELIEFS

Consider some negative or limiting beliefs you may have. They can work well as targets for tapping.

TAKE NOTE

Beliefs are simply ideas you are convinced are true about you, about the world, about men, about women, about health, about work, about food—the list goes on. We are very reluctant to release our beliefs; we feel safe clinging to them because they are so familiar, but they can be deeply damaging to making progress in our lives.

Take the following belief, for example: "I'm too old to lose the weight now." It's important to unpack this belief and how it can affect your success with weight loss. If you are convinced that you're too old to lose weight, the results are simple. You will tell yourself that nothing works, why bother, and you won't even try to lose the weight. And if you start losing the weight, it will contradict your self-image, and you will move heaven and earth to sabotage your success.

What are some other beliefs about you and weight loss that might be blocking your success? Read this list of common beliefs and put a check mark next to any that might be appropriate targets for tapping for you:

- ❑ I'm convinced that nothing will work for me.
- ❑ Everyone in my family is overweight, so I'll always have weight problems.
- ❑ Nothing has ever worked for me before, so why would anything work now?
- ❑ I believe that I have the DNA of a fat person, and nothing can change that.
- ❑ I'm convinced that it gets harder to lose weight every year.
- ❑ I'm convinced that no one has ever been successful with long-lasting weight loss, so why would I be?
- ❑ I'm convinced that it would be dangerous to be thinner.
- ❑ I believe it's not worth the trouble.
- ❑ I'm convinced it's not worth the work I'd have to do.
- ❑ I believe I'm defective and can't succeed.
- ❑ I know my body refuses to lose the weight.

If any of these beliefs sound familiar, then they are worthy targets for your tapping.

TAPPING TARGET: PHYSICAL SYMPTOMS

A final target for tapping can be any of your physical symptoms. These can be related to stress or to being overweight, or they may connect with challenges that make it hard to lose weight. Here are some possible physical symptoms that could be interfering with your success in losing weight:

- ❑ I'm so tired that I need something sugary to pep me up.
- ❑ My joint pain makes everything so hard.
- ❑ I'm exhausted all the time, and I don't feel safe exercising right now.
- ❑ My constant cravings are so distracting all the time, and I don't know how to handle them.
- ❑ My daily cravings make me binge on anything I can get my hands on in the house.
- ❑ My migraines make me want to pull the covers over my head and forget everything.
- ❑ I can't focus well these days, and food helps me concentrate better.
- ❑ I'm feeling weak right now, and eating something makes me feel stronger.
- ❑ My back pain makes it impossible to do anything productive.
- ❑ I'm feeling lethargic, and sugar and caffeine are the only things that make me feel better.
- ❑ I'm feeling physically anxious, and eating calms me down.
- ❑ My arthritis pain makes me forget about healthy eating; I just can't cope.

This first step of tapping is extremely important. If your target doesn't have much punch to it, it won't resonate with you, and reducing the intensity of your feelings about the target won't mean very much. So choose the targets that are really juicy, emotional, and meaningful to you.

While you may have many different targets that you know you need to address in order to stick to a healthy eating plan, I highly recommend that you choose and work on one at a time. Sometimes they feel related—your stress about work triggers cravings for sugar—but address each one separately. You may write a list of your feelings, a list of your beliefs, and a list of your symptoms that all get in the way of your successful weight-loss journey, but if you separate them out and work on one at a time, you will be more successful at reaching your goals.

Sometimes more than one emotion comes up in connection to an event you are tapping about—you might feel resentful that your boss yelled at you and embarrassed when you remember that your coworkers heard him. In this case, it's easy to separate these two feelings into two tapping targets. Work on one at a time until you've reduced your emotional reaction. Then move on to the next target.

The Tapping Diet Method: Step 2

Once you've chosen your target, the next step is to measure how high your discomfort is about the target you've chosen. Using the 0–10 point scale, where 10 is the highest level of distress or anxiety you feel about your situation, consider your target. Are you a 6? A 10? Or only a 4? We take this measurement before and after the tapping so we can determine whether the tapping is working or not. In addition, we often forget how bad our stress was, so having the before and after number is always a good objective measurement.

Some people who are new to tapping feel afraid to choose a target that they know will have a high degree of anxiety or stress attached to it. They'd prefer to start with something smaller and less upsetting. You can choose any targets; however, remember that when you choose a target with an attached stress level of only 3 or 4, it will be harder to feel the effects if it goes down to a 1 or a 2. The tapping will still be effective, but you won't feel the dramatic drop. If you choose stressful targets with distress levels of 7–10, while it might be upsetting at first to focus on them, remember two things:

1. These targets have been there for a long time—they are always operating in your memory anyway, so it's not as if they haven't been bothering you.
2. You will feel great relief in a short amount of time and reduce the feelings quickly and dramatically with the tapping. It's a good idea to practice with a work-related stress, something in the present day, and see how you feel after one or two rounds of tapping.

If you choose a target with a very high level of distress, just know that for decades, practitioners have been using tapping successfully and efficiently to reduce the feelings in a very short period of time. As soon as you start tapping, and as soon as you say the phrase "I deeply and completely accept myself," you will start to feel the distress decreasing. You may also want to add phrases such as "I know the tapping will make me feel better . . ." or "I am happy I finally have a tool to help me feel better . . ." if you are feeling the need for additional reassurance.

Normally, someone's level of distress will decrease during the first round of tapping, in just minutes. That's why this technique has become so popular—it has helped thousands of people reduce their levels of distress in an incredibly short amount of time. Sometimes you need to keep tapping for several rounds on the same topic, and look for one or two underlying layers of feelings about the same topic that might be adding to your distress.

For instance, let's say you are tapping on the resentment about your boss yelling at you. You reduce your resentment from an 8 to a 4 very quickly. You may want to do another round or two of tapping, until this feeling becomes very neutral, and you don't really think about it anymore. Then you move over to the topic of being embarrassed, and you reduce that feeling from a 7 to a 3 very quickly. At that point, you may be reminded of an event where you were yelled at by the coach at school, and so now you have another event and memory of a feeling to tap on . . . but when you look back and measure your feelings about your boss, and about the embarrassment at work, you realize they have continued to go down and feel considerably more neutral. However, now you realize that you need to work on this additional past event, to reduce this feeling of embarrassment from years ago.

So don't be surprised if emotions you've struggled with for years and years go away in just minutes. This is typical and common when working with very clear targets for tapping. Sometimes, an issue feels more stubborn, and you will feel the need to work on it for several days in a row. Other times, there will be several aspects to one topic, and you will feel the need to work on it persistently for a longer period of time. Low self-esteem, for instance, is too broad a topic to tap on—you would need to target specific events, specific phrases that were said to you, your beliefs about having low self-esteem, the evidence you're convinced you have that *proves to you that* you have low self-esteem, etc. This would all take a longer time to release.

The Tapping Diet Method: Step 3

After picking a target and measuring your level of distress over it, the next step is to devise your setup statement. This is a statement that includes a description of the problem (the target) with an affirmation, or a phrase of acceptance. The purpose of this phrase is to reduce your resistance and negativity and prepare you for tapping on the sequence of acupuncture points.

The original phrasing created by Dr. Roger Callahan (who began the tapping movement) is "even though I have this problem [fill in the blank], I deeply and completely love and accept myself."

You can choose a different type of affirmation as long as you remember to use one. One particularly popular variation is called the Choices Method, developed by Dr. Patricia Carrington. Dr. Carrington replaced the classic "I deeply and completely love and accept myself" with phrases that gave the client a choice about how they'd like to feel, such as "even though I feel stressed-out about my job, *I choose to feel* calm and peaceful in this moment." Or "even though I have wild cravings right now and feel out of control, *I choose to feel* calm and satisfied right now."

If you don't like the standard phrase "I deeply and completely love and accept myself," feel free to change it and mix it up, as long as it still feels like you are accepting yourself, your feelings, and your predicament! When you are more comfortable with the basics of the procedure, you will be able to experiment with this part of the setup statement.

TAPPING TIP

Some people find this original setup statement formula a bit too corny for them. If this is the case, I recommend you fish around for another affirmation that you can handle, that you feel comfortable with, even if you take out the "love myself" and just leave in "I deeply and completely accept myself."

Each setup statement includes a description of a target (an emotion, a symptom, a belief, or a memory) combined with an affirmation or statement of acceptance. Read them all out loud so you start to feel comfortable with the rhythm of this all-important part of the tapping procedure.

Once you've done this, take some time to write down some of your own setup statements based on targets you identified in Step 1. Play with this formula until you get comfortable with it, as this will make the process easier. Remember, you are acknowledging the truth about your situation—the truth about your anxiety,

your stress, your hurt, your anger, or whatever you are feeling—
and then adding "I deeply and completely love and accept myself
anyway."

SETUP STATEMENT EXAMPLES FOR GENERAL STRESS

Here are some examples of some setup statements focusing on
general stress. *Remember: when we lose the stress, we lose the cravings
and then the weight!* So if you can address the daily stress in your
life, you can address your lifelong weight problem efficiently and
effectively.

- Even though the stress at work is making me want to over-
  eat right now, I deeply and completely love and accept myself
  anyway.
- Even though I'm distracted by food right now, I accept who I
  am and how I feel.
- Even though I feel stressed-out all over my body, I deeply and
  completely love and accept myself anyway.
- Even though this stress is really getting to me, and I want to
  overeat, I accept who I am and how I feel.
- Even though I feel so stressed I can't concentrate, I accept who
  I am and how I feel.
- Even though I feel so stressed about everything that I can't
  focus, I accept who I am and how I feel.
- Even though my whole body feels stressed-out, I accept who I
  am and how I feel.
- Even though the stress is showing up in my [fill in the blank], I
  choose to love and accept myself anyway.
- Even though the stress is making me hungry all day long, I
  accept who I am and how I feel.
- Even though the stress is triggering my cravings and I can't
  control myself, I deeply and completely love and accept myself
  anyway.

- Even though I can feel myself stress-eating because of this family situation, I deeply and completely love and accept myself anyway.
- Even though my stress is keeping me up at night, I choose to feel calm and peaceful today.

Try coming up with some of your own setup statements that might really resonate with you around how stress shows up in your physical or emotional life. Remember: reducing emotional stress is the key to losing weight successfully. And practicing these statements will help you become more comfortable with the tapping process.

SETUP STATEMENT EXAMPLES FOR CRAVINGS

While we know that stress and worry trigger the hormonal imbalances that lead to food cravings, sometimes we need to address the cravings head-on with tapping. Try saying these statements out loud, and add your own setup statements if my wording doesn't quite match your experiences.

- Even though I'm having these intense cravings right now and I don't know how to control myself, I deeply and completely love and accept myself anyway.
- Even though I want chocolate right this minute, I accept who I am and that I feel out of control.
- Even though I can't control these cravings, I accept who I am and how I feel right now.
- Even though I have to have what I want and I can't wait, I accept who I am and how I feel.
- Even though I feel ravenous and hungry and empty and depleted, I accept who I am and how I feel.

- Even though I feel out of control and have to eat something right now, I deeply and completely love and accept myself.
- Even though I need something to eat to calm me down right now, I deeply and completely love and accept myself anyway.

Again, I highly recommend that you formulate your own setup statements to fit your own cravings. Target how they come over you, how they challenge you, and what you say to yourself when you experience them. You can also address late-night cravings or hunger that seems to hit you out of the blue.

SETUP STATEMENT EXAMPLES FOR FEELING HUNGRY

Here are some examples of setup statements to use when you have the impulse to eat but aren't physically hungry.

- Even though I feel hungry when I know I can't be, I deeply and completely love and accept myself anyway.
- Even though I feel hungry after I just ate, I deeply and completely love and accept myself anyway.
- Even though I'm embarrassed that I feel hungry all the time, I deeply and completely love and accept myself right now.
- Even though it's not possible to be hungry all the time, I choose to accept who I am right now.
- Even though it's frustrating to be hungry in spite of how much I eat, I choose to relax and look deeper at my emotions.
- Even though it's aggravating that I feel hungry all the time, I accept who I am and how I feel.
- Even though I'm afraid to be without food, I deeply and completely love and accept myself.

- Even though not having extra food available makes me feel nervous, I choose to relax and feel back in control.
- Even though there must be something wrong with me because I'm hungry day and night, I deeply and completely love and accept myself.

When we stop and look at our emotions, much of the hunger goes away. What we are truly hungry for is not extra food, but extra love, attention, time, and appreciation. See where in your life you could add some of what you do need, rather than using extra food. If you could get what you needed, would it be food or something more satisfying?

SETUP STATEMENT EXAMPLES OF FEELING HURT

When we feel hurt socially or in our family, if we have been accustomed to reaching for food to anesthetize our feelings, these situations set us up to reach for extra unneeded food. Try these setup statements and add your own that suit your exact situation.

- Even though she said something that really hurt my feelings, I deeply and completely love and accept myself anyway.
- Even though I feel hurt almost every day when someone snubs me, I accept who I am and how I feel.
- Even though I feel hurt by what the team did at work today, I deeply and profoundly love and accept myself anyway.
- Even though I'm way too sensitive, I deeply and completely love and accept myself anyway.
- Even though she hurt my feelings and it makes me want to overeat, I deeply and completely love and accept myself anyway.

Again, try to come up with your own setup statements around this feeling of being hurt, and work on one or two of them a day.

SETUP STATEMENT EXAMPLES FOR FEELING LONELY AND SAD

Loneliness and sadness are emotions many people try to avoid. And what better way to avoid feeling something so unpleasant than reaching for sweet or fatty foods that distract us right away? When we feel lonely or sad, we often feel empty, and filling up with food definitely soothes us from these emotions. Try these setup statements around feeling lonely or sad, and see which ones resonate with you.

- Even though I feel lonely all day long and I can't take it anymore, I deeply and completely love and accept myself.
- Even though I feel lonely and embarrassed about it, I deeply and completely love and accept myself anyway.
- Even though I feel empty inside and just want to eat, I deeply and completely love and accept myself anyway.
- Even though I feel unlovable and fat today, I accept who I am anyway.
- Even though I feel lonely when it's quiet and I know I need to distract myself, I deeply and completely love and accept myself anyway.
- Even though I always reach for food when I feel lonely, I choose to accept myself and my feelings.
- Even though I think I started using food when I was a lonely child, I deeply and completely love and accept myself anyway.
- Even though I feel sad a lot these days, I choose to remember something positive about my life.
- Even though I feel sad about some relationships, I accept who I am and how I feel.
- Even though I feel sad and it makes me want to eat too much, I deeply and completely love and accept myself anyway.
- Even though my sadness overwhelms me sometimes, I deeply and completely love and accept myself right now.

> **TAKE NOTE**
>
> If your sadness seems on the border of depression, please seek professional help and guidance. While EFT may be used as a productive adjunct tool, you need professional help when depression is involved.

Continue coming up with your own setup statements for tapping sequences around the topic of loneliness and sadness. When you're lonely and sad, you feel empty. When you feel empty, you want to fill up with something—anything—and food becomes an easy substitute for companionship.

SETUP STATEMENT EXAMPLES FOR HITTING A PLATEAU

The frustration of hitting a plateau in your weight-loss journey is the kind of emotion that tapping can help you resolve quickly and easily. Use tapping so you don't reach for more food again. Plateaus are an inevitable part of healthy dieting to lose weight, but they are utterly exasperating and tempt people to totally give up. *Don't give up; start tapping!*

- Even though I'm deeply frustrated by hitting a plateau again, I deeply and completely love and accept myself anyway.
- Even though I don't understand why I've hit a plateau again and my weight won't budge, I deeply and completely love and accept myself and my feelings.
- Even though I can't seem to get over this plateau, I choose to accept that I'm still on the right track.
- Even though I feel so frustrated I just want to throw in the towel, I deeply and completely love and accept myself anyway.
- Even though I don't get why this isn't working for me, and I hate hitting this plateau, I deeply and completely love and accept myself anyway.

SETUP STATEMENT EXAMPLES FOR BODY IMAGE

Walking by the mirror can be an unpleasant event and even turn into an emotional battle. When we hate ourselves and our bodies, it creates distressing feelings and subsequent hormonal and endocrine challenges in our bodies, setting us up for wanting more food than we need. Try these statements:

- Even though I really hate my body today, I deeply and completely love myself anyway.
- Even though I don't see how anyone could love me when I'm this fat, I choose to love me anyway.
- Even though I really hate my body and how I look, I choose to find something to appreciate about me.
- Even though I feel embarrassed because I know they're making fun of me, I accept who I am and how I feel.
- Even though I feel ashamed of how I look, I choose to find something good about me now.
- Even though I feel so critical of how I look, I choose to find something good about me now.
- Even though I can't find anything I like about my body today, I choose to accept all of me anyway, no matter what.

Yes, you can learn to appreciate more and more of your body and not use self-hatred as an excuse to reach for extra food when you don't need it. Some people fear that if they like their bodies, they will then relax about their food choices and eat even more! But this is not true. Releasing the self-hatred is the healing you need to stop reaching for unnecessary food.

SETUP STATEMENT EXAMPLES FOR GUILT

When we feel guilty, we tend to feel compelled to punish ourselves. And overeating and breaking our food plan is a great way to punish ourselves, so we can then beat up on ourselves, and start the cycle all over again! Some people feel guilty about things they've said and done in the past; others just feel guilty for not being able to control their eating. Either way, tapping is a superb tool to use on this emotion that can lead you to overeat when you don't need to have any extra food. Try these setup statements:

- Even though I feel guilty for my late-night eating, I accept who I am and how I feel.
- Even though I feel guilty for breaking my diet again, I choose to accept all of me right now.
- Even though I feel guilty for overeating yesterday, I deeply and completely love and accept myself anyway.
- Even though I have some very old guilt that's eating me, I choose to accept who I am and how I feel.
- Even though I think I'm punishing myself because of some very old guilt, I deeply and completely love and accept myself.
- Even though I feel guilty for not being a good enough [choose one: mother, sister, daughter, son, teacher, friend], I deeply and completely love and accept myself anyway.
- Even though I feel anxious about how much guilt I feel, I accept who I am and how I feel.
- Even though I feel guilty about so many things every day, I choose to forgive myself for who I am and how I feel.

So whether you use tapping for guilt about breaking your food plan, or guilt about an incident in your past, it's an excellent tool to help support you and prevent you from abusing food in your life.

SETUP STATEMENT EXAMPLES FOR FEELING UNSAFE

Feeling unsafe in your body can be a primary reason you resist losing the weight, regardless of your caloric intake. If you're feeling unsafe, it won't make sense to you biologically to drop the weight, and your body's wisdom will hold on to every calorie to keep you safe. Try these setup statements and see if any of them resonate for you.

- Even though I feel unsafe in my body, I deeply and completely love and accept myself anyway.
- Even though I don't feel safe in my own body, I choose to feel calm and peaceful anyway.
- Even though I feel unsafe in public, and it makes me want to eat, I deeply and completely love and accept myself no matter what.
- Even though I don't feel safe around men (or women), I deeply and completely love and accept myself right now.
- Even though I feel scared all the time, and it triggers my cravings, I deeply and completely love and accept my thoughts and feelings.
- Even though I feel unsafe in social situations, I deeply and completely love and accept myself and my feelings.
- Even though I can't stand being small, I choose to accept who I am and how I feel.
- Even though I feel so unsafe around other people, so I feel compelled to eat, I deeply and completely love and accept myself and my feelings.
- Even though overeating makes me feel comforted, I accept who I am and how I feel.
- Even though I always think I'm a target for others, I accept who I am and how I feel.
- Even though I feel exposed emotionally and need to keep extra weight on for safety, I accept who I am and how I feel.
- Even though I don't feel safe when I'm smaller, I deeply and completely love and accept myself.

If any distressing memories from childhood come up that you think you could use additional support for, please contact a health-care provider or trained practitioner to help you navigate these safety issues.

CASE STUDY

Jenny never felt safe her entire childhood. She was attacked, abused, ridiculed, and beaten up on a regular basis. She remembers using food to calm herself down and help her feel numb. She said she never really tasted much; it just felt good to be eating. After uncovering why she felt so unsafe, she started to understand why she felt compelled to keep so much extra weight on her body. She admitted that when she was big, she felt like she could ward off her attackers. She felt stronger when she had extra weight on. She felt safer, as if "they" couldn't get to her behind the extra padding. She started to tap on her fear of being attacked, and was able to see that the extra weight was a crutch and didn't do anything real for her. She was able to stop eating so much extra food, and could feel safe again in her own body.

SETUP STATEMENT EXAMPLES FOR FEAR OF LOSING WEIGHT

While we seemed to cover the emotion of fear in the section on feeling unsafe, this language of "fear of losing weight" is more specific, and might resonate even more with you and your situation. Again, if any of these statements feel too uncomfortable and you think you would benefit from additional professional support, please contact a health-care provider or highly trained EFT practitioner for extra support and help.

- Even though I feel afraid every time I lose weight, I choose to calm myself down right now.
- Even though the truth is I'm afraid to lose weight, I deeply and completely love and accept myself anyway.

- Even though I'm afraid to lose weight because I'll feel so exposed, I deeply and completely love and accept all of me.
- Even though losing weight seems dangerous and I no longer feel safe, I accept who I am and how I feel.
- Even though it seems stupid to lose weight because I won't be safe, I accept who I am and how I feel.

When making your setup statements, don't get hung up on perfection or finding the exact right words. Remember to use phrases that sound true to you. Just tell the truth as you tap, and you will be way ahead of the game.

The Tapping Diet Method: Step 4

Once you've chosen your setup statement, repeat it three times while you tap on the first acupuncture point, the karate chop point, located at the base of your pinky finger and above your wrist, on the outside of either hand. Then, you'll tap on a sequence of acupuncture points using a reminder phrase that summarizes what the target is.

Suppose the target for this first round of tapping is "the stress and tension I feel in my body." You would begin by tapping the karate chop point three times while saying, "Even though I feel this stress and tension in my body, I deeply and completely love and accept myself anyway."

Then tap on the sequence of acupuncture points listed while you repeat your "reminder phrase" (for this example, the reminder phrase would be "I feel this stress and tension in my body"). See Chapter 1 for an explanation of the precise location of each acupuncture point.

Decades ago, when Dr. Roger Callahan introduced the tool of tapping to students and laypeople all over the world, each reminder phrase at each point on the face and body was the same. For instance, if you had chosen stress in your body, the reminder phrase would be "this stress in my body" at each of the tapping points.

As the tool of tapping evolved, practitioners started adding variations to the chosen reminder phrase—partly to reduce boredom and habit, and partly to expand on the topic that was chosen. For instance, instead of saying the exact same phrase at each point, which can cause the person to stop paying attention, practitioners would add slight variations, such as "this stress in my body" and "I feel so much stress all over" and "I feel tense from so much stress." The point is not to stray too far from the original reminder phrase, but to be easygoing about what variations you add. If you still feel more comfortable in the beginning just using one phrase at each point, that will of course work! But as an option, and to make it a little more interesting, you can vary each phrase as if you were in a conversation.

The point is to focus on the emotion—and if slightly changing the wording works for you, I highly recommend it. You will see that I change the wording slightly in the following examples, but I am still talking about the exact same target and reminder phrase we originally chose.

While each acupuncture point we are tapping on represents a different organ and emotional challenge in the tradition of ancient Chinese medicine, it's better not to focus on one point corresponding to one emotion. What we are doing is rewiring the energy system, and we are doing this by focusing on a topic and tapping on the entire sequence of energy points.

1. *Eyebrow: I feel this stress and tension in my body*
2. *Side of Eye: My body is so stressed-out*
3. *Under Eye: I feel this stress and tension in my body*
4. *Under Nose: I feel so much stress right now*
5. *Chin: I feel so tense from all the stress*
6. *Collarbone: No wonder I'm having cravings*

7. *Under Arm: I feel so much stress and tension*
8. *Head: Too much stress and tension in my body*

REPEATING STEP 4

If your distress level doesn't go down enough, repeat the tapping. Start with the karate chop point and say, "Even though I feel so much stress and tension in my body, I deeply and completely love and accept myself anyway." Repeat three times.

Now tap on the sequence of acupuncture points listed while you say the reminder phrases that tune you in to the original problem.

Again, notice how I vary the reminder phrases. They all match the situation and target we have chosen to work on, and it often feels really good to say things like "no wonder I want to eat" since that is the truth. And they are all true—the key to your reminder phrases being effective and keeping your attention. Notice that on the eyebrow point, the reminder phrase is "I still feel so much stress and tension" and then down on the collarbone point, the reminder phrase is "I can't relax"—they both are true and both fall under this same category.

Again, it's up to you whether you'd prefer to repeat the exact same reminder phrase on each point, or whether you'd like to vary it according to how you're feeling about the topic. The important thing is that all the phrases are related, and are true for you.

1. *Eyebrow: I still feel so much stress and tension*
2. *Side of Eye: All this stress and tension in my body*
3. *Under Eye: I feel so much stress and tension*
4. *Under Nose: No wonder I want to eat*
5. *Chin: There's too much stress and tension in my body*
6. *Collarbone: I can't relax*
7. *Under Arm: Too much stress and tension*
8. *Head: I feel exhausted from all this stress and tension*

You can continue as needed.

Of course you can do a tapping exercise with stress as your target several times a day. This is an excellent exercise to do, especially at the end of the day when you've left work, but you've taken the emotions of the job home with you!

The Tapping Diet Method: Step 5

The next step is to take another measurement of your distress level when you consider your target. Remember to use the 0–10 point scale. Has your distress level decreased significantly? If not, do another round of tapping with the target in mind. Then check again. It may take several rounds of tapping to reduce your distress level about the target.

That's it! The process of tapping, once you become familiar with it, is really quite straightforward and easy to do. It will quickly become a very powerful tool for you in your weight-loss challenge.

CHAPTER SUMMARY

In this chapter:

- We discussed how using tapping can help you deal with emotions connected to feelings of deprivation, weight-loss plateaus, and many other problems.
- We looked specifically at each of the steps in *The Tapping Diet* method, including choosing a target, measuring your level of distress, creating a setup statement, performing the tapping, and measuring your level of distress again.
- We covered scripts to help you identify targets and create useful setup statements.

CHAPTER 4

KEEP ON TRACK WITH YOUR DAILY TAPPING PLAN

In Chapter 2, you learned why tapping is such a spectacular tool for weight loss, and in Chapter 3, you were given information on how to specifically use the tapping method to lose weight.

Now, in this chapter, you'll put it all together by creating a simple, doable daily plan. Remember: the best routine is one that you will actually follow. It can't be too complicated, too long, or too hard to complete. The point of a daily tapping plan is to reduce your overall emotional stress. This tapping plan will reduce your cravings, and stop the automatic behavior of reaching for food when you feel strong emotions, such as fear, loneliness, resentment, or frustration. If your plan becomes an additional cause of stress, that defeats its purpose.

This chapter also includes a number of scripts you can use to deal with particularly thorny issues that may be getting in the way of your success in achieving your weight-loss goals. (Chapter 5 has even more scripts for you to use.)

▶ PUT IT ON YOUR CALENDAR

I highly recommend a specific tapping plan for my coaching clients, or else the tapping won't get done during the day. It will simply fall off your to-do list. When you're not feeling in crisis, and your days are going along well enough, you don't feel the need for support tools. This is a serious problem, because as you know, you can often be going along just fine and then wham! The cravings hit you, or some unexpected stress comes at you from your boss or the kids, and you resort to your old habits of using food to soothe yourself.

This is why a plan is so important. It takes care of what actually drives the cravings in the first place, and soothes those moments of stress and your emotions before they gain momentum and you feel out of control.

Consider different times of the day that would be ideal for tapping. If you can tap during a few of those times, great! Even better if you can tap during *all* of those times—that would be ideal and speed up your progress.

TAPPING TIP

Think about what times of day you feel vulnerable to overeating, times when the stress is high, your cravings are high, or there is ample opportunity to cheat on your diet. These times are often in the morning, before lunch, during midafternoon, after work, before dinnertime, and late at night.

Choose at least twice a day where you put aside the time for your tapping. I urge you to carve out this time and respect and protect it. There is no room during these times for dogs, kids, telephones, or computers, just quiet space for you and your tapping assignments. If you tap more often, you will reduce more of your stress, the culprit behind your overeating.

TAKE NOTE

The point of tapping during the day rather than waiting for an emergency is that regular tapping will calm down your overall anxiety and stress, and allow you to handle feelings that trigger your overeating. Don't wait until you're in the car on your way to Dunkin' Donuts to tap—you simply won't do it!

▶ SAMPLE TAPPING PLAN: MORNING

Let's walk through a sample tapping plan so that you can see what I mean about creating a daily action plan. Let's start with first thing on a Monday morning:

You've had a good weekend; you're feeling calmer after a chaotic week last week; and you're tempted to skip your stress-relief tapping. You imagine your boss has had the weekend to calm down, too, about all the deadlines, and you're maintaining your healthy eating plan. But you notice a mild concern surfacing as you picture yourself walking back into the office. You know the stress at work triggers your cravings and overeating. Nothing feels urgent but maybe this would be a good time to tap for a couple of minutes.

Yes, even though you don't feel urgent and nothing is boiling over, this is exactly when you need to do your tapping!

Choose a target—something that's bothering you, an anticipated stressor, a mild concern about sticking to your diet, or something you think could trigger you when you get to the office—and start tapping. (Don't choose some upsetting event from your past; those topics are better dealt with when you have a safe period of time to focus at home.)

Sample Script for Tapping

Use the Monday-morning scenario to practice tapping.

Step 1. Choose your target. In this case, your target is "I'm slightly agitated about going back to work."

Step 2. Measure the intensity of the feeling on the 0–10 point scale. Since we're considering this a mild stressor, it's probably a 4 or 5 on the scale.

Step 3. Create a setup statement. "Even though I feel agitated and a little stressed because I don't know what mood my boss will be in, I deeply and completely love and accept myself anyway."

Step 4. Tap on the acupuncture points. Starting by tapping on the karate chop point, say your setup statement three times. Then, move through the sequence:

1. *Eyebrow: I feel slightly anxious about going back to work.*
2. *Side of Eye: I feel nervous . . . I don't know what I'll be facing.*
3. *Under Eye: What if my boss is in a bad mood again?*

4. *Under Nose: I feel that slight anxiety.*
5. *Chin: I'm concerned about the mood in the office.*
6. *Collarbone: What if things hit the fan again?*
7. *Under Arm: I'm worried about what the mood will be.*
8. *Head: I'm starting to feel concerned about sticking to my diet.*

Step 5. Measure your distress level. Take a deep breath and consider the level of stress you feel about going back to work, using the 0–10 point scale. Hopefully it has decreased, but you may be more aware than ever that you do get triggered by other people in the office. I recommend tapping for one or two more rounds on this worry. This will allow you to start your day feeling peaceful and calm, no matter what *they* do in the office.

Round Two Script

While tapping on the karate chop point, say the setup statement: "Even though I'm still a little worried that work will be chaotic again, I deeply and completely love and accept myself anyway." Repeat three times. Then, go through the tapping sequence:

1. *Eyebrow: What if work is crazy like last week?*
2. *Side of Eye: I barely stuck to my eating plan last week.*
3. *Under Eye: I'm worried I'll overeat because of my nerves.*
4. *Under Nose: I have no idea what's going to come at me.*
5. *Chin: I hate not knowing.*
6. *Collarbone: It makes me nervous.*
7. *Under Arm: I'm worried about the unknown.*
8. *Head: I feel my anxiety rising right now.*

Take a deep breath, and measure your anticipatory stress/anxiety again on the 0–10 point scale.

These exercises will get you to the office in a calm, peaceful state, no matter what your boss or coworkers are doing! Start your day out right, and it will unfold more smoothly for you from every angle.

It's important to take the time to check in with your feelings, and tapping first thing in the morning, or before you go to work, will smooth out your emotions for your entire day. Even if you're not in danger of relapsing on your diet plan, you will feel much better physically and emotionally, and will probably be better able to concentrate and do a good job.

▶ SAMPLE TAPPING PLAN: NOON

Now it's lunchtime—you waited a little long, so you feel ravenous. You're not sure if you're feeling true body hunger or if some of the stress from your morning is making you hungrier than usual. This would be a great time to stop and tap for a few minutes to calm yourself down so you don't eat for the wrong reasons. Unfortunately, what usually happens is that you are not aware of your stress levels or emotions that have surfaced during the morning, and instead of stopping to notice or become aware of them, you use food to quiet them down and get instant relief. That's why so many people eat more than they intend to. They aren't paying attention to why they're eating so fast and so much.

Again, the tapping isn't supposed to suppress a real appetite, but it will reduce the stress and anxiety that tends to cause us to eat more than necessary.

Sample Script for Tapping

Step 1. Choose your target. In this case, your target is "I feel starving and want to eat anything and everything right now."

Step 2. Measure this feeling on the 0–10 point scale. It may seem challenging to stop and tap when you're hungry, but the two minutes of tapping will do wonders for reducing your appetite and improving your mood.

Step 3. Create a setup statement. "Even though I feel starving, and I just want to eat something to feel relief, I deeply and completely love and accept myself anyway."

Step 4. Tap on the acupuncture points. Starting by tapping on the karate chop point, say your setup statement three times. Then, move through the sequence:

1. *Eyebrow: I feel starving and want to eat everything in sight.*
2. *Side of Eye: I feel so hungry I can't concentrate.*
3. *Under Eye: I feel starving.*
4. *Under Nose: I'm so hungry I could eat anything.*
5. *Chin: I feel starving right now.*
6. *Collarbone: I wonder how much of this is from the stress.*
7. *Under Arm: I feel so hungry right now.*
8. *Head: I'm starving, even though I ate breakfast a few hours ago.*

Step 5. Measure your current distress level. Take a deep breath and measure your hunger again using the 0–10 point scale. The tapping won't take your hunger away, but it will take the edge off that feeling of starving.

Round Two Script

If you could tap for one more round, you would greatly calm yourself down, and then make better food choices for lunch.

While tapping on the karate chop point, repeat the setup statement: "Even though I still feel starving, and I could eat anything, I deeply and completely love and accept myself." Repeat three times, then move into the acupuncture sequence.

1. *Eyebrow: I'm still so hungry.*
2. *Side of Eye: I want to eat everything in sight!*
3. *Under Eye: I'm still way too hungry.*
4. *Under Nose: I'm starving right now.*

5. *Chin: I wonder how much stress is affecting me.*
6. *Collarbone: So much stress today.*
7. *Under Arm: No wonder I'm so hungry.*
8. *Head: I want to calm myself down right now.*

Take a deep breath, and measure your ravenous hunger again on the 0–10 point scale. You may still be hungry, but it's unlikely that your hunger feels out of control. With a couple of tapping sequences under your belt, you will be able to eat a normal-sized meal, slowly and pleasurably, and feel calm and settled when you go back to work.

▶ SAMPLE TAPPING PLAN: AS NEEDED

If at any time during your day, at home or at the office, you feel mildly upset or irritable, it's a great time to use tapping to take the edge off the emotions and calm yourself down. Even if you're not in danger of overeating at these times, the tapping will do wonders and last throughout the rest of your day. Remember: the stress and unchecked emotions are what make you reach for more food than you need. We'll do a round of tapping that sounds more general. If at any time you'd like to change the wording to better suit your situation, please do.

Sample Script for Tapping

Step 1. Choose your target. In this case, your target is "I feel unsettled and unfocused."

Step 2. Measure this feeling on the 0–10 point scale.

Step 3. Create a setup statement. "Even though I feel unsettled and unfocused, I deeply and completely love and accept myself anyway."

Step 4. Tap on the acupuncture points. Starting by tapping on the karate chop point, say your setup statement three times. Then, move through the sequence:

1. *Eyebrow: I feel kind of unsettled emotionally.*
2. *Side of Eye: I'm not really sure what's going on.*
3. *Under Eye: I feel a little unsettled and unfocused.*
4. *Under Nose: I know that eating would make me feel better.*
5. *Chin: But I don't want to eat anything right now.*
6. *Collarbone: I feel unsettled emotionally.*
7. *Under Arm: I feel kind of hungry right now.*
8. *Head: I want to eat to take the edge off of my feelings.*

Step 5. Measure your current distress level. Take a deep breath and feel this emotion on the 0–10 point scale again. Where are you now? I know feeling unsettled is uncomfortable, and not knowing exactly what you're feeling is a true setup for you to use food to make you feel numb. Just stopping momentarily, checking in with yourself, and asking yourself what you are feeling can slow down the automatic reaction to reach for food. And when you slow down, you can think about it consciously and change your behavior patterns.

Round Two Script

You may find that another round of tapping would help settle your discomfort.

While tapping on the karate chop point, say the setup statement: "Even though I still feel unsettled, I deeply and completely love and accept myself." Repeat three times. Then go through the sequence of acupuncture points:

1. *Eyebrow: I have a lot going on and feel unsettled.*
2. *Side of Eye: I feel unsettled with everything that's going on.*

3. *Under Eye: I feel unsettled.*
4. *Under Nose: I feel agitated and unsettled.*
5. *Chin: I have lots of feelings and it would be easier to overeat.*
6. *Collarbone: I feel unsettled and want to calm down.*
7. *Under Arm: I choose to calm down.*
8. *Head: I want to feel calmer.*

Take a deep breath and measure this feeling again on the 0–10 point scale. If any specific instances from your day come up, you can go ahead and plug those in to the tapping sequences and do a couple more rounds. You will definitely feel calmer and better able to handle what's going on, and as a result, you won't use so much food to quiet yourself down.

▶ SAMPLE TAPPING PLAN: AFTER WORK

Now it's that vulnerable time after work and before dinner—a dangerous time for people who use food to calm down their feelings. You're feeling tired from your day, and you're a little hungry but not quite ready for dinner. Sometimes people have other tasks to do at this time, with the kids or laundry or cleaning up, and eating can be a good distraction!

Try to tune in to your emotions at this time of day. How are you feeling? What's happening in your mind? Are you exhausted and want to overeat? Irritated and want to erase the feelings from the day?

Sample Script for Tapping

Step 1. Choose your target. In this case, your target might be something like "I'm exhausted from the day and want a reward."

Step 2. Measure how true this feels on the 0–10 point scale.

Step 3. Create a setup statement. "Even though I feel emotionally and physically exhausted and want a reward, I deeply and completely love and accept myself anyway."

Step 4. Tap on the acupuncture points. Starting by tapping on the karate chop point, say your setup statement three times. Then, move through the sequence:

1. *Eyebrow: I feel mentally exhausted and want a reward.*
2. *Side of Eye: I feel tired on all levels and feel I deserve a reward.*
3. *Under Eye: I feel exhausted and resentful.*
4. *Under Nose: I did way too much today.*
5. *Chin: I'm exhausted and need a reward.*
6. *Collarbone: I'm really exhausted and want to eat right now.*
7. *Under Arm: I want to overeat to shut out my hard day.*
8. *Head: I want to overeat to be quiet and calm.*

Step 5. Measure your level of distress again. Take a deep breath, and consider your level of mental and/or physical exhaustion. How does your body feel? How does your mind feel? Hopefully you are feeling calmer and better able to handle your emotions. And now you won't need to use food to calm yourself down—you can use tapping instead!

Round Two Script

Try one more round for your emotional and physical feelings at this time of day.

While tapping on the karate chop point, say the setup statement: "Even though I feel washed out and exhausted, I deeply and completely love and accept myself." Repeat three times. Then go through the sequence of acupuncture points:

1. *Eyebrow: I still feel exhausted.*
2. *Side of Eye: I feel washed out.*

3. *Under Eye: I know some sugar would help me right now.*
4. *Under Nose: I could use a pick-me-up.*
5. *Chin: I'm exhausted on all levels.*
6. *Collarbone: I just want to zone out.*
7. *Under Arm: I'm exhausted mentally and physically.*
8. *Head: I just want to numb myself right now.*

Take a deep breath and measure your emotional and physical exhaustion again—hopefully it's gone down enough that you can now make intelligent food choices. You don't need to eat something you'll regret later, and you don't need to eat quickly and mindlessly.

CASE STUDY

Fran reported that she would feel slightly unsettled and agitated at the end of her day. She'd come home at 5:30 P.M., take the dog for a walk, read the mail, and then have nothing to do. She said she would feel increasingly unsettled with the quiet and stillness in her house. She would often resort to raiding the pantry even though she was planning a regular dinner shortly. With exploration and some tapping, she finally understood that this unsettled feeling was from her fear that in the quiet times, old emotions from childhood sometimes surfaced. They were very confusing and extremely unsettling. And overeating immediately shut them down. After endless cycles up and down on the scale, she finally asked for support with a tapping practitioner and was able to heal these emotional conflicts from her past and stop using food as a way to shut up these emotions.

At this time if you have the privacy, you might want to target an emotion or even a memory that is bigger than just the leftover feelings from your day. Maybe there's a bigger theme going on for you that comes from a relationship, or your family—something that would be worth tapping on that keeps you feeling low or unworthy. See Chapter 5 for additional scripts you might use for other emotions.

▶ SAMPLE TAPPING PLAN: DINNERTIME

Now it's dinnertime. You're naturally hungry, but a little too stressed-out, and you suspect you might overeat during this meal. Start tapping to calm yourself down so you can eat slowly and mindfully.

Step 1. Choose your target. In this case, your target might be something like "I feel the urge to overeat."

Step 2. Measure how true this feels on the 0–10 point scale.

Step 3. Create a setup statement. "Even though I feel the urge to overeat at dinner, I deeply and completely love and accept myself anyway."

Step 4. Tap on the acupuncture points. Starting by tapping on the karate chop point, say your setup statement three times. Then, move through the sequence:

1. *Eyebrow: I want to blot out the day.*
2. *Side of Eye: Finally, I get a reward.*
3. *Under Eye: I have this urge to overeat.*
4. *Under Nose: I want to reward myself with food.*
5. *Chin: I have a lot of emotions from the day.*
6. *Collarbone: I don't know what to do with them.*
7. *Under Arm: I have so many emotions from the day.*
8. *Head: Dinner would make me forget everything.*

Step 5. Measure your level of distress again. Take a deep breath and measure your urge to overeat on the 0–10 point scale.

Round Two Script

Keep tapping until the urge to overeat goes down so far, you are just looking forward to a normal meal that will be pleasurable and satisfying.

While tapping on the karate chop point, say the setup statement: "Even though I have this urge to overeat, and I can feel it coming on, I deeply and completely love and accept myself anyway." Repeat three times. Then go through the sequence of acupuncture points:

1. *Eyebrow: I have this urge to overeat.*
2. *Side of Eye: This urge to overeat.*
3. *Under Eye: My urges are so strong.*
4. *Under Nose: This urge to overeat now.*
5. *Chin: I want to blot out the day.*
6. *Collarbone: This strong urge to overeat.*
7. *Under Arm: I can feel it right now.*
8. *Head: This strong feeling of wanting to overeat.*

Take a deep breath and enjoy the calm coming over you from the tapping. You can now have a good healthy dinner, eat slowly, and feel satisfied without needing to overeat.

▶ SAMPLE TAPPING PLAN: LATE EVENING

Many people tell me they feel lonely at night, and use this time to overeat to calm themselves down. Does that sound like you?

Sample Script for Tapping

Step 1. Choose your target. In this case, your target might be something like "I feel lonely and alone and want to use food to feel better."

Step 2. Measure the intensity of this feeling on the 0–10 point scale.

Step 3. Create a setup statement. "Even though I feel lonely and alone and want to use food to feel better, I deeply and completely love and accept myself anyway."

Step 4. Tap on the acupuncture points. Starting by tapping on the karate chop point, say your setup statement three times. Then, move through the sequence:

1. *Eyebrow: I feel lonely late at night.*
2. *Side of Eye: It's too quiet and I want to overeat.*
3. *Under Eye: I feel lonely and alone.*
4. *Under Nose: I want to overeat.*
5. *Chin: I feel so lonely.*
6. *Collarbone: It makes me want to overeat.*
7. *Under Arm: I feel lonely and alone.*
8. *Head: I want to overeat.*

Step 5. Measure your level of distress again. Take a deep breath and measure your feeling of loneliness again on the 0–10 point scale.

Round Two Script

You might find the urge to overeat going down, but you might still feel lonely. Tap another round for this emotion.

While tapping on the karate chop point, say the setup statement: "Even though I still feel lonely, I deeply and completely love and accept myself anyway." Repeat three times. Then move through the sequence of acupuncture points:

1. *Eyebrow: I still feel lonely and alone.*
2. *Side of Eye: I hate this feeling.*
3. *Under Eye: No wonder I overeat late at night.*

4. *Under Nose: I feel so alone.*
5. *Chin: I feel alone and lonely and want to use food.*
6. *Collarbone: I feel alone and lonely.*
7. *Under Arm: I have urges to overeat when I feel lonely.*
8. *Head: I feel alone and lonely.*

Take a deep breath and measure your feeling of loneliness again. Hopefully you feel calmer and better able to handle this emotion, so you don't need to resort to overeating.

Since you have some time before going to bed, it's another segment in your day where you might be drawn to work on a deeper issue in your life, rather than the stress from your day.

Is there a relationship that needs some healing? A betrayal from someone that still stings? Fear of being exposed if you lose the weight? A safety issue? Spend some time tapping to release these emotions.

▶ SAMPLE TAPPING PLAN: BEDTIME

It's bedtime! This is another good time for you to use tapping to release the stress from your day. Whether your stress came from work, your family, or circumstances outside in your environment, you deserve to be able to release them and let go so you can enjoy a peaceful, deep sleep. When you sleep better, your body feels safer and doesn't need to hold on to extra weight. When you sleep well, your hormones have a chance to even out more, and you don't need to hold on to extra calories to maintain your feeling of safety.

Sample Tapping Script

Step 1. Choose your target. In this case, your target might be something like "I feel anxious about going to sleep; there's too much to worry about."

Step 2. Measure how high this level of stress feels to you on the 0–10 point scale.

Step 3. Create a setup statement. "Even though I feel anxious and don't want to go to sleep, I deeply and completely love and accept myself anyway."

Step 4. Tap on the acupuncture points. Starting by tapping on the karate chop point, say your setup statement three times. Then, move through the sequence:

1. *Eyebrow: I feel anxious and don't want to fall asleep.*
2. *Side of Eye: I feel all this leftover stress.*
3. *Under Eye: I want to release this stress and sleep well.*
4. *Under Nose: I want to feel relaxed before going to bed.*
5. *Chin: I choose to release my stress.*
6. *Collarbone: I love feeling better about releasing my stress.*
7. *Under Arm: I choose to feel lighter and happier.*
8. *Head: I love releasing the stress from my day.*

Step 5. Measure your level of distress again. Take a deep breath, and measure your level of anxiety on the 0–10 point scale. Again, consider whether this is a safety issue, and whether you feel the need to be alert and awake instead of peaceful and asleep. See Chapter 5 for sample scripts on tapping for safety issues.

Round Two Script

You may find that another round or two of tapping will help you relax enough to fall asleep without anxiety and tension.

While tapping on the karate chop point, say the setup statement: "Even though my head is buzzing from all the emotions during the day and I can't calm down, I deeply and completely love and accept myself anyway." Repeat three times. Then move through the sequence of acupuncture points:

1. *Eyebrow: I can't calm down.*
2. *Side of Eye: I feel kind of hyper.*
3. *Under Eye: Food would help me calm down.*
4. *Under Nose: I feel anxious about so many things.*
5. *Chin: I choose to feel calm right now.*
6. *Collarbone: Lots of leftover feelings and anxiety.*
7. *Under Arm: Lots of extra emotions from the day.*
8. *Head: I choose to release them now.*

Take a deep breath, and enjoy the feelings of peace and calm as you allow yourself to slip off into a very deep and peaceful sleep.

TAPPING TIP

If, during the day, other specific emotions surface, like resentment or fear, turn to Chapter 5 for more scripts on how to tap on those feelings.

If you approach your day and life as if you deserve to release your stress (and you know that stress will always be around because we all have lives, families, jobs, and our health to worry about), you will be way ahead of the game. Tap with the purpose of releasing your excess stress, and soon you will be feeling better in all areas of your life. Most importantly, you will feel healthier mentally and emotionally, and you won't feel the need to reach for food that isn't healthy or necessary.

▶ CREATE YOUR OWN DAILY PLAN

Using the information given in Chapter 3, identify a few targets that you plan to work on in the immediate future. Create a script that you can use that feels right and authentic to you (see Chapter 5 for additional sample scripts).

PERSONAL SCRIPT

Target: _____

Setup Statement: _____

1. *Phrasing for Eyebrow Tapping:* _____
2. *Phrasing for Side of Eye Tapping:* _____
3. *Phrasing for Under Eye Tapping:* _____
4. *Phrasing for Under Nose Tapping:* _____
5. *Phrasing for Chin Tapping:* _____
6. *Phrasing for Collarbone Tapping:* _____
7. *Phrasing for Under Arm Tapping:* _____
8. *Phrasing for Head Tapping:* _____

Then, as suggested earlier in this chapter, consider times of the day when you are more likely to feel stressed, overwhelmed, or tired—at risk of overeating even if you're not physically hungry. Then make a plan, listing times of day that you plan to tap, and the target you plan to tap on. Keep in mind that you can change this target if the day brings up a different emotion or situation that you want to tap on. Then, use the plan to record your level of distress after each tapping round. Here's a template you can use:

DAILY TAPPING PLAN				
TIME OF DAY	TARGET	LEVEL OF DISTRESS	# OF TAPPING ROUNDS	REMEASUREMENT OF DISTRESS

▶ OTHER STRATEGIES TO SUPPORT YOUR TAPPING PRACTICE

There is no doubt that the tool of tapping is exceptional for helping you reach your weight-loss goals. If you create a daily plan and follow it, you'll increase your chances of success to a significant degree.

In Chapter 5, I provide more tapping scripts to help you deal with stressors and emotions that may be making your weight-loss journey more challenging. But there are also other practices I recommend to help you stay on track while moving toward your weight-loss goals. I encourage you to consider adding some or all of these additional practices to your repertoire. After all, any additional support you can get is good for you! Imagine how much progress you could make if you added more support tools to your life.

People often feel as if food is being taken away from them, as if dieting is a punishment. Their sense of deprivation is very real, especially if they don't have the emotional resources to deal with the emotions that they are using food to numb. Whenever you can *add* something into your day, rather than taking something away, that will help your overall stress levels and emotional balance. Some of my favorite strategies are journal writing, mindfulness, meditation, and creative visualization. Let's dig into each of these a little further to see how they can support your tapping efforts and help you on your weight-loss journey.

Journal Writing

A time-honored tradition for support, journal writing is incredibly effective for releasing pent-up emotions. You can act as if you're writing out your emotions to yourself, to a higher self, to the divine, to nature, or just to free the space in your mind by getting them out of your head and onto a blank page.

I would have to say that 100 percent of the people I know who use a journal for extra support love this process, and find solace and comfort in the daily practice. You don't need to be rigid and journal every single day, but I recommend you use journaling to get clarity on your feelings and emotional conflicts. This will reduce your stress levels and ultimately help you on your weight-loss journey.

TAKE NOTE

Science is showing the multiple health benefits from journal writing. It appears to lower our stress levels and help us feel calmer, regardless of what's going on in our lives. Journaling can be so flexible, and it's a wonderful way to share your feelings without being judged by anyone. It's known as a method to improve your insight, increase your personal growth, and improve your ability to resolve emotional conflicts from work or home. In addition, journaling can help you develop self-compassion.

There is no right or wrong way to journal. You can use it just to process the events of the day, or to record positive things that have happened, or in any number of different ways. However, one way to get started is to use the tapping targets you've identified as a way to prompt some reflection about your emotions or about past events. You can use journaling to help untangle a complicated experience so that you can develop specific targets to tap. You can use journaling to get to the bottom of what's really eating you.

See the section called "An Attitude of Gratitude" for ways to keep a gratitude journal.

Mindfulness

Much has been written about positive studies involving mindfulness, which can work to calm the nervous system and boost positive hormones and feelings. Mindfulness is simply a way of going about daily activities with a sense of awareness. Have you ever had the experience where you've driven home from work and don't remember a single thing about the trip? That experience of being on autopilot is the exact opposite of what we are trying to accomplish with mindfulness. Experts recommend that you make an effort to be attentive, focused, and clear about exactly what you are doing in the moment. Multitasking is a no-no as it diverts your concentrated attention.

What does mindfulness have to do with weight loss? Remember that feeling stress is counterproductive for our physical bodies, our emotions, and our habits. When we feel stress, not only do our hormones react; we tend to forget to do what's good for us (tapping, walking, journaling), and we tend to lean toward unhealthy behaviors again (overeating).

So when you learn how to use mindfulness throughout the day, you are remembering what's good for you. You're aware of your stress levels, which means you are improving your chances of remembering to do your tapping, improving the even flow of your hormones, reducing cravings, and feeling better in general!

Remember earlier when I talked about how sometimes your cravings can get so overwhelming that you find yourself eating without having even stopped to think about tapping? Mindfulness is a method you can use to help ensure that you do the tapping when you need to.

TAKE NOTE

Mindfulness is used as a therapeutic technique and requires focusing your awareness on the present moment while accepting your feelings and bodily sensations instead of judging them. *Psychology Today* describes a mindfulness practice as "living in the moment and awakening to experience." Researchers and practitioners such as Jon Kabat-Zinn have established specific programs using mindfulness and meditation to reduce overall stress.

Meditation

While mindfulness and meditation have a lot in common (people who practice one usually practice the other), meditation is a specific practice that you set aside time to do, whereas mindfulness is more of an attitude.

During your busy day, taking a few minutes for meditation practice is like giving yourself a gift—a gift of quiet, relaxation, and peace. We all need more peace in our lives, and the more peaceful we are, the more centered we are. And the more centered we are, the better able we are to stick to our goals, and follow the path to healthy weight loss! Meditation can be directly useful to and supportive of any weight-loss program you are on. Meditation has been shown to lower our overall stress levels, and since stress is a clear target when reducing cravings and overeating, reducing those stress levels reduces your likelihood of having cravings and overeating.

Some people find it helpful to use guided meditation recordings to help them meditate. Personally, I prefer to be quiet rather than listening to a premade audio recording of someone else's voice, but it is totally up to you. A meditation practice that works is one that you take time to do. Take simple steps, don't overwhelm yourself, and make sure to schedule time for meditation into your day.

MEDITATION BASICS

Here are some basic steps that will help you establish a meditation practice.

- Choose a time of day that works well for you. (I can't meditate before bed because I invariably fall asleep. Sleep is fine, but it's not meditation.)
- Choose a comfortable place where you can sit or lie down.
- Eliminate distractions. Turn off your phone, let the dog out, and close down your computer.

- Focus on your breathing, in and out, in and out. You may count your breaths if this helps you stay more focused. You may also choose a specific calming word, such as "peace" or "love," to focus on if this helps you stay focused. You might repeat your chosen word ("mantra") on each out breath.
- There's no need to be perfect; just the fact that you have made an effort to meditate is a win for you in your life.
- Set a timer, and once or twice a day, complete a five-minute meditation.

MEDITATION SCRIPT

Here is a sample meditation script. You can record these words and play them back when you set aside your meditation time.

1. Get yourself comfortable in a sitting position, and notice how your body feels. Notice the support behind your back, your hips, and how your feet feel on the floor. Notice your posture, and how comfortable you feel being quiet, and notice what it feels like when you breathe, in and out, in and out.

2. Now notice the temperature in the room, what the temperature feels like on your face, on your skin, around your body. And take another deep breath in and out. Notice how the air feels filling your lungs, and notice what it feels like to exhale, slowly and completely.

3. Notice your thoughts as they move through your mind and choose to let them go. Accept that you have these thoughts moving in and out, in and out, as your breathing goes in and out, in and out. Accept and notice your thoughts and then let them go, one by one.

4. Now notice what sounds you hear in the room, and what sounds you might be hearing coming from outside. Let these sounds move in and out of your awareness, fading into the background, coming

forward again, fading again out of your awareness. Just allow them to help you go deeper and deeper into a peaceful place of awareness and calm.

5. Enjoy feeling so calm and peaceful. Enjoy feeling quiet and calm. Notice your breathing and how peaceful and rhythmic it feels, in and out, in and out. Notice the stillness. Notice how good you feel when you are quiet and still, quiet and still, as your breathing slows down and feels calm and peaceful, calm and peaceful.

6. Notice how quiet you feel, how peaceful you feel, and how still your body and mind feel right now. Enjoy the quiet and peace of mind, knowing that you are doing something so healthy for yourself, breathing in and out, quiet and calm, relaxed and peaceful.

7. And when you feel ready, you can take a deep breath, open your eyes, and get reoriented to your time and place, and feel calm, relaxed, and rejuvenated from the quiet stillness in your body and mind.

Creative Visualization

Visualization exercises are different from basic meditations in that they are specifically focused on reaching a chosen goal. During meditation you are supposed to just relax and feel peaceful without doing anything; in a visualization exercise you are supposed to act as if you have reached a specific goal.

- Choose a specific goal you would like to reach in your life. Then formulate a successful vision of this completed goal as if you have already attracted it into your life. To support a weight-loss goal, imagine that you have already achieved success.
- You can complete visualizations for many different parts of your life. But separate them at first so you aren't feeding your mind too much information and getting confused. In other words, start with your weight-loss goal; then later you can add

a financial success goal; then later add the imagery of a successful relationship; and so on.

- Once you have chosen your specific goal, start adding the tex-
  ture of your senses. Notice how it looks now that you have
  arrived at this end result. What do you see from your eyes
  now that you have reached your goal? What do you see in
  your external world? What scenery? What reflections in the
  mirror? How are people looking at you now that you have
  been successful?
- Feel how it *feels* physically to be successful in reaching this goal.
  Notice how you feel in your body; notice your posture, how
  your gait feels, how your muscles feel now that you have successfully reached your goal. Act as if you are already there, and
  enjoy the physical sensations.
- How do you feel emotionally now that you have reached your
  goal? Feel the confidence, the happiness, the joy, the peace of
  mind. Act as if you are already there, and notice your emotional
  mood, what feelings are coming up, what's new and enjoyable
  now that you have reached your goal.
- Notice any smells or tastes associated with your success. Flow-
  ers of congratulation? Perfume? Fresh air as you're able to be
  more active?

CASE STUDY

Jessie, one of my clients, does a few minutes of tapping before she enters
into a meditation. She feels it calms her down and centers her so that she
can be more peaceful and quiet during her short meditation.

During her meditation, she uses creative visualization to tap on
herself while in this state of meditation. She says she feels calm and
quiet, and uses her imagination to tap on the tapping points. Again,
she picks a simple target, taps slowly and methodically in her mind on
the points, while saying the reminder phrases in her mind, and feels

completely relaxed and peaceful when her meditation ends. She says it's better to do short meditations this way; otherwise she gets distracted. She reports that this practice helps her feel calm and neutral about food—when she might normally feel hungry, she doesn't, and during times that are challenging for her when cravings surface, she no longer struggles with these cravings.

A note about visualization and tapping: In the previous case study, I mentioned Jessie, who uses tapping in her mind while she meditates. Many people need to use visualization as a way to tap when they are in public. For instance, I have a client in New York who has a phobia about entering a crowded subway car—yet she needs to do that every day to get to work! I taught her to look in the mirror while she tapped, so she knew what it looked like. She would do a few rounds of tapping at home before she had to leave, choosing targets such as "I'm afraid to be around crowds" and "I don't like being squished" and "I feel out of control in the subway." Then while she was actually on the subway train, she would close her eyes and mentally go through a few rounds of tapping. She would tap physically on her karate chop point because no one would notice that, but then she would tap in her mind on the points on her face and body while mentally repeating her reminder phrases.

This way, no one thought she was strange or weird, and she was able to calm herself down considerably before getting to work. She said that not only did it greatly reduce her fear of being on the subway; when she followed this practice, her overeating would drop dramatically during the day. She suspected that tapping on her anxiety during the ride to work calmed her down in general, and she didn't feel the need for extra food to calm her down when she got to work.

An Attitude of Gratitude

When we focus on an attitude of gratitude, everything can change for the better. Our usual self-talk involves self-criticism, mean commentary, disgust, self-loathing, and other unfriendly language that our bodies and minds are required to absorb. When you're in the middle of that nasty scolding or commentary, you can't help but take it in. So what if you turned this perspective around, stopped hating your body, and started appreciating you, your body, your strength, and who you are?

I know what would happen. You would feel better, lighter, more present, and happier in general. And when you're happier in general, you are less likely to let all that stress get to you and sabotage your health and weight-loss plans. When you have more compassion for yourself (a common end result of the mindfulness and meditation practices listed), you tend to take better care of yourself. And when you are inspired to take better care of yourself, it will show up in how, when, and what you eat. People who feel inspired to take care of themselves don't eat junk food several times a day; it is no longer congruent with their self-image. Having a food binge no longer feels right when you are taking care of and loving your body, your mind, and your spirit.

So my prescription to combat the chronic negative self-talk we are all involved in is to write a general gratitude list every day. You may write this list in the morning or at night, whichever feels better to you. The steps are simple, but the results can be miraculous. Here are some steps to take to cultivate an attitude of appreciation.

RECORD YOUR THOUGHTS

Buy a small, colorful notebook that looks pleasing, fun, and pretty to you. This is a sacred place where you'll write your appreciation and grateful thoughts.

KEEP A LIST

Every day, write out ten things you feel grateful for. They don't need to be huge items. They can be very simple. ("I feel grateful I got the laundry done this weekend.")

CHANGE IT UP

Change the title of your list for some variety. Here are some options that will trigger the feelings of gratitude, optimism, and appreciation, all of which will help raise your vibration and your mood:

FIVE THINGS I LOVE ABOUT MY LIFE

1. I love my work schedule right now
2. I love my new neighbor
3. I love how I'm cooking healthy food for myself
4. I love feeling supported by my meditation practice
5. I love my friendships

FIVE THINGS I LOVE TO DO

1. I love eating healthy meals
2. I love taking long, relaxing walks
3. I love writing in my journal
4. I love listening to uplifting music
5. I love browsing in a bookstore

FIVE THINGS I LOVE ABOUT MY BODY

1. I love how strong my legs are
2. I love the shape of my face
3. I love that I have such sharp eyesight
4. I love my smile
5. I love that my eyes and my child's eyes are the same

FIVE THINGS I'M GRATEFUL FOR TODAY

1. I'm grateful I woke up on time
2. I'm grateful I was prepared for work
3. I'm grateful I have easy transportation
4. I'm grateful I'm healthy
5. I'm grateful I'm a fast thinker

You get the point! When you focus on gratitude and look for reasons to be grateful in your life, you will be amazed at what positive experiences show up for you. Try these simple writing exercises to support your emotional journey, and you will love the return on your investment in terms of peace, calm, and happiness.

My clients have regularly told me that keeping a gratitude journal has helped them reduce cravings, improve how they feel about themselves, and decrease their overeating in general. One client even said she made a gratitude list about how much she had learned about herself regarding her overeating tendencies. Normally she would have made a mental list of everything she did wrong, but when she learned about making gratitude lists, it really helped her focus and viewpoint. All of the gratitude practices helped her to accept herself more, to reduce her self-criticism, and to keep her more on track when she followed a healthy eating plan.

CHAPTER SUMMARY

In this chapter:

- We described the importance of following a daily action plan in order to get the most from *The Tapping Diet.*
- We went through a sample day, step by step, with sample scripts that you can use.
- We provided a sample template for you to use to create your own daily plan.
- We explored several additional support tools to help you on your weight-loss journey, including journaling, mindfulness, meditation, and creative visualization.

CHAPTER 5

SAMPLE SCRIPTS FOR TAPPING

You may discover that various issues crop up as you continue your weight-loss journey. You may reduce your distress over one target only to find that it was really covering for something else. For example, the memory of a past experience may bring up a number of related emotions, and you may need to tap separately for these emotions. It can be helpful to have specific scripts that will guide you through tapping for each of these issues. That's what you'll find in this chapter.

Once you've gone through these tapping scripts a few times, you may find that you're ready to develop your own scripts that deal more specifically with your targets and with your authentic reactions to those targets. Or, you may wish to continue using the provided scripts. Either approach is fine—it's up to you.

▶ ADDITIONAL TAPPING SCRIPTS

In this chapter, you will find tapping scripts that deal with the following feelings:

- anxiety
- cravings
- guilt
- loneliness
- hurt
- anger
- resentment
- safety issues
- deprivation
- unworthiness

Each sample script includes at least one example of a second-round script you can use to further reduce your level of distress surrounding each emotion. The language for these second-round scripts is slightly different to reflect that you have already gone through one round of tapping.

Tapping on Anxiety

When we feel anxious, it can be about something specific, like the deadline your boss gave you, or it can feel free-floating and not connected to anything. Since it's hard to put your finger on free-floating anxiety, it can be hard to know how to alleviate it. Unfortunately, eating does wonders to soothe your anxiety. It is both distracting and biologically calming. Heavy foods, such as carbohydrates and sugars, have a sedating effect, so you may have been treating your anxiety all these years without knowing how to calm down on your own.

Tapping is a superb tool to use to help you calm down without the use of outside substances. Follow the usual five-step method you were shown in Chapter 3.

Step 1. Choose your target. In this case, your target might be "I feel so anxious all the time."

Step 2. Measure how anxious you feel now, about a particular topic or in general, using the 0–10 point scale.

Step 3. Create a setup statement. "Even though I feel so much anxiety in my life, every day, I deeply and completely love and accept myself anyway."

Step 4. Tap on the acupuncture points. Starting by tapping on the karate chop point, say your setup statement three times. Then, move through the sequence:

1. *Eyebrow: I feel so anxious all the time.*
2. *Side of Eye: I don't know how to calm myself down.*
3. *Under Eye: I feel so anxious all the time.*
4. *Under Nose: I don't even know why I'm so anxious.*
5. *Chin: I feel so anxious and eating helps me feel better.*
6. *Collarbone: I feel so anxious all the time.*

7. *Under Arm: I know that eating soothes me.*

8. *Head: I want to feel calm on my own.*

Step 5. Measure your distress again. Take a deep breath and measure your anxiety level on the 0–10 point scale. Hopefully it has gone down a few points. But I highly recommend tapping on this topic again. Here's a script for round two:

Start by tapping on the karate chop point, using your setup statement: "Even though I still feel anxious in my body and mind, I deeply and completely love and accept myself anyway." Repeat three times. Then, move through the sequence:

1. *Eyebrow: I feel so anxious all the time.*

2. *Side of Eye: I really feel anxious and uncomfortable.*

3. *Under Eye: I feel so anxious.*

4. *Under Nose: I feel so anxious.*

5. *Chin: I feel anxious and jittery.*

6. *Collarbone: I feel uncomfortable and want to overeat.*

7. *Under Arm: I feel so anxious.*

8. *Head: I really feel anxious.*

Take a deep breath and measure your anxiety level on the 0–10 point scale again. Tap a few more rounds on this topic if necessary.

Tapping on Cravings

Now let's say you are really struggling with cravings, and while you know that the cravings feel physical, they come up because of tension or stress or anxiety. When this is the case, you can't focus on your emotions because the cravings feel too urgent for you and you just know you're going to eat something that's not good for you or will take you down the wrong road.

Step 1. Choose your target. In this case, your target might be something like "these intense cravings I have."

Step 2. Measure how high your cravings are right now on the 0–10 point scale. If they were a 10, you probably already ate something, but if you're trying to avoid overeating, you may be able to wait and tap before running for the fridge.

Step 3. Create a setup statement. "Even though I have these intense cravings right now, I deeply and completely love and accept myself anyway."

Step 4. Tap on the acupuncture points. Starting by tapping on the karate chop point, say your setup statement three times. Then, move through the sequence:

1. *Eyebrow: These intense cravings.*
2. *Side of Eye: I don't think I can resist them.*
3. *Under Eye: These intense cravings.*
4. *Under Nose: I want what I want right now!*
5. *Chin: I don't know how to resist.*
6. *Collarbone: It feels good to acknowledge my intense cravings.*
7. *Under Arm: But I don't think I can resist them.*
8. *Head: And that's okay, too.*

Step 5. Measure your level of distress. Now take a deep breath, and measure your intense cravings again on the 0–10 point scale. Where are your cravings now? Lower, I hope. But go ahead and do at least one more round of tapping on the cravings until you feel confident you can resist them and move on with your day. Here's a script for round two:

Start by tapping on the karate chop point and saying, "Even though I can still feel my intense cravings right now, I choose to feel calm and peaceful." Repeat three times, then go through the acupuncture sequence:

1. *Eyebrow: I still have these intense cravings.*
2. *Side of Eye: How am I going to resist?*

3. *Under Eye: These intense cravings.*
4. *Under Nose: I want to eat something right now.*
5. *Chin: I feel agitated by my cravings.*
6. *Collarbone: I wish I could feel calm instead.*
7. *Under Arm: These intense cravings.*
8. *Head: I want to eat something right now.*

Take a deep breath and measure the level of your cravings again on the 0–10 point scale. Hopefully, your cravings have gone down significantly, and you can resist eating those tempting foods when you're not hungry. If you want to do another tapping round to get the cravings even lower, go ahead. And if you suspect a particular emotion is driving your cravings, use this emotion as the target in your next tapping sequence.

TAPPING TIP

Please note that when the cravings dissipate, sometimes the real emotions that were fueling the cravings surface. So if you've tapped these past two rounds, and your cravings went down, you might feel other emotions that were the cause of your cravings. Go ahead and plug those feelings in as your new tapping target, and proceed as described until the emotion subsides dramatically.

Tapping on Guilt

When we feel guilty about something we said or did, or didn't say or didn't do, we tend to punish ourselves. It's just how the brain and human nature works. So I would like to lead you through a tapping sequence to reduce your overall guilt.

Step 1. Choose your target. In this case, your target might be something like "I feel guilty because I overate yesterday."

Step 2. Measure how high this feeling of guilt rates on the 0–10 point scale.

Step 3. Create a setup statement. "Even though I feel guilty because I overate yesterday, I choose to forgive myself and move on."

Step 4. Tap on the acupuncture points. Starting by tapping on the karate chop point, say your setup statement three times. Then, move through the sequence:

1. *Eyebrow: I feel so guilty about breaking my diet.*
2. *Side of Eye: I feel so guilty about what I ate yesterday.*
3. *Under Eye: I keep beating myself up for overeating.*
4. *Under Nose: I can't stand that I sabotaged myself.*
5. *Chin: I feel so guilty.*
6. *Collarbone: I want to give up.*
7. *Under Arm: I'm mad at myself and feel so guilty.*
8. *Head: I feel guilty and can't believe I broke my diet.*

Step 5. Measure your level of distress again.

In addition to feeling guilty about breaking your diet, some of you may feel guilty about other things in your life. Some of you may think you should feel guilty, and you don't want to forgive yourself. That's up to you. But remember: intense emotions make us overeat, and make us hold on to extra weight. So I highly recommend following this next exercise on guilt for your round two tapping session. Here you'll choose a slightly different target, along the lines of "I feel guilty about something from my past [fill in the blank here for what you feel guilty about]."

Start by tapping on the karate chop point and saying your setup statement: "Even though I feel guilty about something I did in the past, I deeply and completely love and accept myself anyway." Repeat three times. Then follow the acupuncture sequence:

1. *Eyebrow: I feel so guilty about that past incident.*
2. *Side of Eye: I can't believe I said/did what I did.*
3. *Under Eye: I feel so guilty about that incident in my past.*

4. *Under Nose: I feel so guilty and I can't seem to get over it.*
5. *Chin: I'm not sure I want to get over it.*
6. *Collarbone: I think I should feel guilty; I did something wrong.*
7. *Under Arm: I should feel guilty and I should be punished.*
8. *Head: I wish I didn't feel this way.*

Take a deep breath and, while thinking of the same incident you chose for this tapping round, measure how guilty you feel on the 0–10 point scale. Hopefully, your guilt has gone down a lot. If not, you can continue to tap on this incident. Here's a sample of what your round-three script could sound like:

Start by tapping on the karate chop point and saying your setup statement: "Even though I still feel guilty for what I did back then, I deeply and completely love and accept myself anyway." Repeat three times. Then go through the sequence of acupuncture points:

1. *Eyebrow: I still feel guilty.*
2. *Side of Eye: I shouldn't have done it.*
3. *Under Eye: I still feel guilty.*
4. *Under Nose: I wonder if I am punishing myself with sabotage.*
5. *Chin: I still feel guilty.*
6. *Collarbone: I still blame myself.*
7. *Under Arm: I wonder if I'm ever going to let this go.*
8. *Head: I still feel so guilty, but will consider letting it go.*

Take a deep breath, and measure how guilty you feel again on the 0–10 point scale. Hopefully, your guilt about this specific incident has gone down dramatically.

TAKE NOTE

After you've been tapping for a while, you will notice a difference in how you treat yourself. You will be more compassionate, and have fewer reasons to beat up on yourself. Remember: when you feel compelled to beat up on yourself, reaching for food when you're not hungry sounds like a good idea in the moment.

Tapping on Loneliness

Now let's move on to another emotion: loneliness. Everyone feels lonely at different times in their lives, but if overeating is a problem for you, it's likely that loneliness fuels this behavior.

Step 1. Choose your target. In this case, your target might be something like "I feel lonely and empty and I eat because of it."

Step 2. Measure how true this feels to you on the 0–10 point scale.

Step 3. Create a setup statement. "Even though I feel lonely a lot and overeat because of this, I deeply and completely love and accept myself anyway."

Step 4. Tap on the acupuncture points. Starting by tapping on the karate chop point, say your setup statement three times. Then, move through the sequence:

1. *Eyebrow: I feel lonely and empty.*
2. *Side of Eye: I've always felt lonely and empty.*
3. *Under Eye: Food helps me to feel full and satisfied.*
4. *Under Nose: I feel so lonely and empty.*
5. *Chin: I'm afraid to feel these feelings so I overeat.*
6. *Collarbone: I hate feeling lonely and empty.*
7. *Under Arm: I usually overeat to feel better.*
8. *Head: I feel lonely and empty a lot.*

Step 5. Measure your level of distress again. Take a deep breath and measure your feelings of loneliness and emptiness again.

Hopefully, the pain of these feelings has decreased. I recommend tapping on this topic again. Here's a sample script for a second round of tapping:

While tapping on the karate chop point, say the setup statement: "Even though I still feel lonely and empty inside and it makes me overeat, I deeply and completely love and accept myself anyway." Repeat three times. Then, move through the sequence:

1. *Eyebrow: I still feel lonely.*
2. *Side of Eye: I still feel empty inside.*
3. *Under Eye: No wonder I'm so focused on food.*
4. *Under Nose: I feel lonely and empty.*
5. *Chin: I hate feeling so empty.*
6. *Collarbone: I use food to fill me up, but it doesn't work.*
7. *Under Arm: I use food to fill up my emptiness.*
8. *Head: I'm tired of overeating when I feel lonely and empty.*

Take a deep breath and measure your feeling of loneliness and emptiness again on the 0–10 point scale. You may continue tapping on this topic if it resonates deeply with you, and certainly return to these tapping scripts during your week if you suspect these feelings trigger you to overeat.

Tapping on Hurt

Let's tap on hurt, a powerful feeling from our past and our present that can trigger us to use food to avoid the pain.

Think of an incident when you felt hurt, from your recent history or from your past. It's very uncomfortable, isn't it? That's your clue that you may be overeating to ignore the pain or avoid going there.

Step 1. Choose your target. In this case, your target might be something like "I still feel hurt by what happened."

Step 2. Measure how hurt you feel on the 0–10 point scale. This may surprise you, especially if the incident is from a long time ago.

But this hurt festering inside can lead you to use food to distract yourself.

Step 3. Create a setup statement. "Even though I still feel hurt by that past incident, I deeply and completely love and accept myself anyway."

Step 4. Tap on the acupuncture points. Starting by tapping on the karate chop point, say your setup statement three times. Then, move through the sequence:

1. *Eyebrow: I feel hurt when I think of that incident.*
2. *Side of Eye: I can't believe it still hurts me.*
3. *Under Eye: It was a long time ago, but it still hurts.*
4. *Under Nose: I think I've been trying to avoid it.*
5. *Chin: Overeating helps me ignore this past hurt.*
6. *Collarbone: It still really stings, all these years later.*
7. *Under Arm: I still feel really hurt.*
8. *Head: And I think I'm using food to avoid feeling my hurt.*

Step 5. Measure your level of distress again. Take a deep breath, think of the incident, and measure how hurt you feel now on the 0–10 point scale. Proceed with another tapping round on the target of feeling hurt, and then change to other incidents if you have several of them that need to be cleared. Here's a possible script for a second round of tapping:

While tapping on the karate chop point, say the setup statement: "Even though I still feel hurt when I think of what happened, I deeply and completely love and accept myself anyway." Repeat three times. Then, move through the sequence:

1. *Eyebrow: I still feel hurt when I think of what happened.*
2. *Side of Eye: It wasn't fair.*
3. *Under Eye: I still feel hurt.*
4. *Under Nose: It still stings when I think about it.*

5. *Chin: I'd like to let it go.*
6. *Collarbone: It's been bothering me for so long.*
7. *Under Arm: It's time to let it go.*
8. *Head: I feel better already.*

Tapping on Anger

Now let's move on to another strong emotion that can cause you to reach for food when you're not even hungry: anger. Most people don't want to feel their anger. They haven't had good models in their life of what it looks like to be and feel angry without attacking, criticizing, or blaming, so it's a very unpleasant emotion.

TAKE NOTE

Eating can certainly block your feelings, particularly anger. Some people don't even think they have any anger, but when they stop using food as anesthesia, they realize they've been covering anger for decades.

There is nothing wrong with feeling angry, but you must not hurt someone else because of it. Anger isn't bad, but hitting someone because you're angry is not acceptable.

Take a person you're angry at, and make a tapping target out of this scenario:

Step 1. Choose your target. In this case, your target might be something like "I feel angry when I think of my [mother, father, brother, sister, colleague]."

Step 2. Measure how angry you feel when you think of this person, using the 0–10 point scale.

Step 3. Create a setup statement. "Even though I feel angry when I think of that person in my life, I deeply and completely love and accept myself anyway."

Step 4. Tap on the acupuncture points. Starting by tapping on the karate chop point, say your setup statement three times. Then, move through the sequence:

1. *Eyebrow: I really feel angry at her/him.*
2. *Side of Eye: I am surprised at how angry I feel.*
3. *Under Eye: I really feel angry at him/her.*
4. *Under Nose: I wonder if I'm overeating because of my anger.*
5. *Chin: I really feel angry at this person.*
6. *Collarbone: I feel angry whenever I think of her/him.*
7. *Under Arm: No wonder I try to avoid this person!*
8. *Head: I really feel angry and think I've been overeating because of it.*

Step 5. Measure your level of distress again. Take a deep breath and measure how angry you feel now on the 0–10 point scale. I know nothing changed—that person is still that person and still did what they did to make you angry—but measure the intensity of your anger. Hopefully, it has already gone down in just one round. I recommend tapping again on this topic. Here's a possible script for a second round of tapping:

While tapping on the karate chop point, say the setup statement: "Even though I still feel angry and I'm not sure I want to give it up, I deeply and completely love and accept myself." Repeat three times. Then go through the sequence of acupuncture points:

1. *Eyebrow: I still feel angry at him/her.*
2. *Side of Eye: I still feel angry.*
3. *Under Eye: I think I've been overeating to avoid the anger.*
4. *Under Nose: This makes a lot of sense to me now.*
5. *Chin: I still feel angry, but not as much.*
6. *Collarbone: I should be angry.*
7. *Under Arm: But I'm willing to let it go.*
8. *Head: I still have some anger left, and that's okay, too.*

Take a deep breath and measure how angry you feel on the 0–10 point scale. Make sure you do not switch targets—make sure you are measuring your anger about the same person or incident right now. You can always tap on your anger about another person or incident at a later time.

Tapping on Resentment

Now let's talk about resentment. Resentment is a powerful emotion that you might feel entitled to have, given what someone did to you; however, it's one of those emotions that totally fuels you to overeat. So it is really worth tapping on any resentments you are holding on to.

Step 1. Choose your target. In this case, your target might be something like "I feel resentful about [fill in the blank]."

Step 2. Measure how resentful you feel about what happened on the 0–10 point scale. Don't be surprised if you are all the way up at a 10! This happens easily, and when we feel justified, we don't want to let this feeling go. But I am certain you can understand how resentment can get in the way of an easy weight-loss journey.

Step 3. Create a setup statement. "Even though I feel so resentful about this issue, I deeply and completely love and accept myself anyway."

Step 4. Tap on the acupuncture points. Starting by tapping on the karate chop point, say your setup statement three times. Then, move through the sequence:

1. *Eyebrow: I am full of resentment.*
2. *Side of Eye: I can't believe I still feel resentful.*
3. *Under Eye: I feel so resentful right now.*
4. *Under Nose: I thought this was in the past.*
5. *Chin: I feel so resentful.*
6. *Collarbone: It feels hard to let it go.*

7. *Under Arm: I don't want to let it go.*
8. *Head: I feel really resentful about what happened.*

Step 5. Measure your level of distress again. Take a deep breath and measure this resentment on the 0–10 point scale. Another angle might surface, but stay focused on the resentment, and tap again. Here's a sample script you might use:

While tapping on the karate chop point, say your setup statement: "Even though I feel eaten up by my resentment, I deeply and completely love and accept myself anyway." Then, move through the sequence:

1. *Eyebrow: I feel so resentful.*
2. *Side of Eye: I'm surprised at how resentful I feel.*
3. *Under Eye: All this resentment is eating me up alive.*
4. *Under Nose: All this resentment.*
5. *Chin: I feel so resentful.*
6. *Collarbone: I want to let it go.*
7. *Under Arm: It's hard to let it go.*
8. *Head: All this resentment.*

Take a deep breath and measure your level of resentment again on the 0–10 point scale. Keep tapping with resentment as your target until these past incidents no longer have a charge for you. Then you know you can be free of these emotions and conflicts, and it will be easier to stick to a healthy eating plan.

Tapping on Safety Issues

If you don't feel safe losing the weight, it doesn't really matter what you eat because out of survival tactics, your physical body will hold on to every calorie and keep you the same size it thinks you need to be for emotional or physical safety. Not only can tapping on safety help you feel better every day of the rest of your life; it will help you lose the weight, and your body and mind will be getting the right messages now—that you are safe, and that you don't need the extra weight for protection.

Step 1. Choose your target. In this case, your target might be something like "I feel unsafe without the extra weight as protection. I'm afraid to lose the weight."

Step 2. Measure your level of distress on the 0–10 point scale. You can measure this two different ways: Either measure how true this statement feels to you ("I feel unsafe"), or measure how afraid you would feel when you picture or imagine yourself without the extra weight.

Step 3. Create a setup statement. "Even though I'm afraid to lose the extra weight, I deeply and completely love and accept myself anyway."

Step 4. Tap on the acupuncture points. Starting by tapping on the karate chop point, say your setup statement three times. Then, move through the sequence:

1. *Eyebrow: I'm so afraid to lose the weight.*
2. *Side of Eye: I need my extra protection.*
3. *Under Eye: I'm so afraid to be smaller.*
4. *Under Nose: It doesn't feel safe to lose the weight.*
5. *Chin: I'm afraid to be without my protection.*
6. *Collarbone: My weight and size make me feel safer.*
7. *Under Arm: I'm afraid to lose the weight.*
8. *Head: I didn't know I felt so unsafe without the weight.*

Step 5. Measure your level of distress again. Take a deep breath and measure your fear again on the 0–10 point scale, or your level of feeling unsafe without the weight. Don't make this an intellectual exercise; make it come from your gut. This topic always needs several rounds of tapping. And as I mentioned earlier, if you need to seek additional professional help, please do so for these safety issues. A possible script for a second round of tapping is this:

While tapping on the karate chop point, say your setup statement: "Even though I still don't feel safe when I think of losing the weight, I deeply and completely love and accept myself anyway." Repeat three times. Then go through the sequence of acupuncture points:

1. *Eyebrow: I still don't feel safe without my weight.*
2. *Side of Eye: I want this extra protection.*
3. *Under Eye: I feel the need for the extra protection.*
4. *Under Nose: I want my extra weight.*
5. *Chin: No wonder I've been struggling to lose weight.*
6. *Collarbone: A part of me doesn't want to lose it.*
7. *Under Arm: No wonder I go up and down.*
8. *Head: I'm afraid to lose the weight.*

Now let's tap for a positive round—for the first fifteen years of tapping, no one made any positive suggestions, but practitioners started adding positive statements, and they became very popular. Now I think it's a good idea for this topic. (Feel free to add a round of positive statements to any of your tapping sequences.) While tapping the karate chop point, say a positive setup statement, like "even though I haven't felt safe in the past without my extra weight, I choose to feel safe now." Continue to tap on the sequence of points, saying these positive phrases:

1. *Eyebrow: What if I could feel safe now?*
2. *Side of Eye: What if I could feel safe even without the weight?*
3. *Under Eye: I choose to feel safe without the weight.*
4. *Under Nose: I love feeling safe, now that I'm an adult.*
5. *Chin: I choose to be safe now.*
6. *Collarbone: I don't need this extra weight anymore.*

7. *Under Arm: I appreciate what my body's been trying to do for me.*
8. *Head: I choose to feel safe without all the extra weight.*

Here's another script you can use for a positive round of tapping:

1. *Eyebrow: It feels good to feel safe now.*
2. *Side of Eye: I didn't used to feel safe.*
3. *Under Eye: I like feeling safer now.*
4. *Under Nose: I can handle my feelings when I'm smaller now.*
5. *Chin: I appreciate my body and that it can keep me safe.*
6. *Collarbone: I appreciate feeling safe now.*
7. *Under Arm: I love feeling safe.*
8. *Head: I deserve to feel safe now.*

Tapping on Deprivation

What about feeling deprived? You may feel as if you want more food, but what do you really feel deprived of in your life?

Step 1. Choose your target. In this case, your target might be something like "I feel deprived of love and attention."

Step 2. Measure your level of distress. How deprived do you feel, using the 0–10 point scale?

Step 3. Create a setup statement. "Even though I feel deprived of love and use food to fill the hole, I deeply and completely love and accept myself anyway."

Step 4. Tap on the acupuncture points. Starting by tapping on the karate chop point, say your setup statement three times. Then, move through the sequence:

1. *Eyebrow: I feel deprived and use food instead.*
2. *Side of Eye: I have felt deprived as long as I can remember.*
3. *Under Eye: I feel so deprived.*
4. *Under Nose: I want more of something . . . love and attention.*

5. *Chin: No wonder I overeat.*

6. *Collarbone: I need love, not food.*

7. *Under Arm: I need love and attention, but I don't have enough.*

8. *Head: I feel so deprived.*

Step 5. Measure your feelings of distress again. Take a deep breath and measure how deprived you feel now on the 0–10 point scale. You may have gained insight into a more specific feeling of deprivation, or recalled memories of events that happened when you were a child that caused you to feel deprived. You can tweak the language and continue tapping. Here's a sample script for a second round of tapping:

While tapping on the karate chop point, say the setup statement: "Even though I have always felt deprived of love from my mother, I deeply and completely love and accept myself anyway." Repeat three times. Then go through the sequence of acupuncture points:

1. *Eyebrow: I never got enough attention from her.*

2. *Side of Eye: I always felt deprived of love and attention.*

3. *Under Eye: No wonder I use food to feel better.*

4. *Under Nose: Overeating works temporarily.*

5. *Chin: I feel deprived of love from my mother.*

6. *Collarbone: I feel so deprived.*

7. *Under Arm: I feel so deprived of love and attention.*

8. *Head: No wonder I've been using food to fill the emptiness.*

Take a deep breath and measure this feeling of deprivation again on the 0–10 point scale. I hope it makes sense why food is an easy crutch when you feel deprived of love and attention. You can be starving for love, and reach for food, even though it is only a short-term fix.

Mary felt deprived of love, time, attention, and food her whole life. She was one of many siblings, and there never seemed to be enough time or attention to go around. She was sandwiched somewhere in the middle of a lot of kids, and never felt that her parents had any time left by the time she came around. In addition, money was very tight in her family, and she described lots of control issues with her parents. They started locking the pantry so the kids couldn't get extra food. Mary said they were never starving, but there was barely enough, and they would have enjoyed extra snacking in the evenings. So when Mary grew up, she started eating whatever she wanted whenever she could, just to combat this feeling of deprivation. She knew it didn't make sense, but she didn't want to give up her newfound freedom. Once she tapped on the feeling of deprivation from childhood, she could eat when she chose to, not just because she could! She was able to lose the extra weight, feel much more relaxed at meals, and feel satisfied in new ways.

Tapping on Feelings of Unworthiness

Suppose you have been told or you believe you have low self-esteem. The important question is: "How do you know you have low self-esteem?" Many people answer that they know they have low self-esteem because they feel unworthy when they're with their peers, or they don't feel deserving of success. If this is the case, you can try these tapping rounds, and remember to be as specific as possible. "I have low self-esteem" is not a specific enough target, but "I feel unworthy whenever I think of reaching my goals" is.

Step 1. Choose your target. In this case, your target might be something like "I feel unworthy when I think of reaching my goals."

Step 2. Measure your level of distress. How unworthy do you feel, using the 0–10 point scale?

Step 3. Create a setup statement. "Even though I feel unworthy whenever I think of moving ahead, I deeply and completely love and accept myself anyway."

Step 4. Tap on the acupuncture points. Starting by tapping on the karate chop point, say your setup statement three times. Then, move through the sequence:

1. *Eyebrow: I feel unworthy and less than.*
2. *Side of Eye: I feel unworthy when I think of reaching my goals.*
3. *Under Eye: What's the point?*
4. *Under Nose: Why bother?*
5. *Chin: I don't think I'm worth it.*
6. *Collarbone: I think I was taught that.*
7. *Under Arm: They taught me I wasn't worth it.*
8. *Head: I don't feel worthy of reaching my goals.*

Step 5. Measure your level of distress again. Take a deep breath, and consider how unworthy you feel, using the 0–10 point scale.

It's worth noting that, if you do in fact feel unworthy or *less than*, you had to learn that somewhere. Some authority figure or parent or teacher had to communicate that to you with either his behavior or her words. This would be a time, if you feel safe enough, to go deeper with your tapping and to try to understand and work on one of these negative lessons you learned in childhood. Here's a sample script for round two:

While tapping on the karate chop point, say the setup statement: "Even though I felt unworthy because there was never enough for me as a kid, I deeply and completely love and accept myself anyway." Repeat three times. Then go through the sequence of acupuncture points:

1. *Eyebrow: I felt left out and unworthy.*
2. *Side of Eye: No one paid attention to me.*

3. *Under Eye: No wonder I don't think I'm worth it.*
4. *Under Nose: I always feel unworthy.*
5. *Chin: There was never enough attention or love for me.*
6. *Collarbone: I always feel unworthy.*
7. *Under Arm: I don't think I'm worth it.*
8. *Head: I feel unworthy.*

Take a deep breath, and measure this feeling of unworthiness again on the 0–10 point scale. Do you need some more rounds of tapping? Do you need to write out some of your thoughts and feelings? Remember to be very specific when you use these topics for tapping. "Low self-esteem" is too broad a topic, but "I feel unworthy whenever I'm with other people" is a great tapping target.

CASE STUDY

My client Penny told me she had felt lonely most of her life. She said she felt unworthy socially, physically, and emotionally, and never felt like she was worth attention from anyone. Her parents were preoccupied with work and their own fighting, so being quiet and invisible worked for Penny as a child. In her silence, she learned how to resort to food for comfort.

Penny had an impression that her mother offered her too many sweets and too much food on a regular basis because it made her feel like a good mother who was providing for her daughter. The truth is, Penny needed love and undivided attention, not food. Once this became clear to Penny—that she had been given food instead of love and attention as a child—she had some significant insights into her behavior. She was able to stop criticizing herself as much and used tapping in very productive ways. She tapped on feeling empty; she tapped on feeling unworthy of attention; and she tapped on feeling lonely as a kid.

She started to notice when she felt real hunger instead of just eating all the time out of habit. She started to adjust how much she ate, how often she ate, and what kinds of foods she ate. She noticed that she actually wanted more fruits and vegetables, and that while eating a lot of junk food was a habit, it didn't taste that good to her. Penny was very consistent with her tapping, even between our sessions, and learned how to address her stress and the cravings that came up when she felt unworthy. She was able to lose weight, but much more importantly, she felt better about herself, felt lovable and worthy, and started to value who she was in the world. She even forgave her parents for their lack of attention, and realized it was their issue, not a reflection of her worth.

CHAPTER SUMMARY

In this chapter:

- We explored a number of sample scripts that show how to use tapping to deal with many common emotions that create difficulties for people on their weight-loss journey.
- We looked at round-two scripts that alter the language slightly for subsequent tapping rounds.
- We learned how to specifically use tapping to deal with anxiety, cravings, guilt, loneliness, hurt, anger, resentment, safety issues, deprivation, and feelings of unworthiness.

PART 2

INTRODUCTION TO HEALTHY EATING

Now that you know how to use tapping to focus on and release the emotional reasons you overeat, it's time to take a look at information that can help ensure that you're putting the best into your body. Even though changing your diet isn't the biggest thing you can do to lose the weight, nurturing yourself and your body with good-for-you foods with a low calorie count will help you on your journey. In Chapter 6, you'll learn the basic of healthy eating and in Chapter 7, you'll find fifty healthy recipes that will work to support your weight-loss goals.

CHAPTER 6

THE BASICS OF HEALTHY EATING

While you may often hear the word "diet" used in a negative way, or a way that makes you cringe, the real, deep-down meaning of the word (and a much more positive one) is anything that you eat or drink for nourishment. Eating the right diet to provide your body with the nutrients it needs also ensures that you are eating the right diet to manage your weight . . . assuming you are staying within your caloric needs.

In this chapter you will learn about the important changes that you should make to your diet and receive info on what foods you should be eating regularly to provide good nutrition to your body.

▶ WHAT DO YOU NEED TO KNOW?

The more you know about nutrition, the better—but you don't need to be a trained expert to understand the basic principles to keep yourself lean and healthy. Some foods are better than others, and this depends on the amount of desirable nutrients (or nutrient density) that they provide per serving. Some nutrient-dense foods include:

- Fruits and vegetables in a variety of colors, which are packed with antioxidants and fiber.
- Whole-grain, fiber-filled foods like brown rice, whole-wheat bread, whole-wheat pasta, oats, barley, and quinoa (there are many others).
- Lean proteins, like fish, white-meat poultry, lean cuts of meat, legumes, eggs, low-fat dairy, and soy.
- Foods containing omega-3 fatty acids, such as fish, flaxseed oil, canola oil, soybeans, pumpkin seeds, and walnuts.
- Nutrient-rich foods, which are those foods packed with many vitamins and minerals in each serving.

Other foods to limit that provide very few of the nutrients you need include:

- Foods containing saturated fats, which are found in fatty cuts of red meat, cheese, full-fat dairy products, and fried food.
- Foods containing trans fats, which are formed when oils are altered to be solid and can be found in margarines, many baked goods (especially if they are not homemade), and fast foods.
- Refined grains like white rice, white bread, and "wheat" bread that is not 100 percent whole grain.
- Nutrient-poor foods, which are those that are high in calories per serving, don't provide many desirable nutrients, and often contain saturated fats and added sugars.
- Overly processed, prepackaged foods containing saturated fats and added sugars.
- High-sodium foods.
- Beverages with added sugars—particularly sodas and some juices—as these pack in the calories but not the vitamins and minerals (and you won't get the benefit of fiber when drinking juice).

And, while everyone needs a different amount of calories each day, the basic nutrition guidelines *guide* you toward making the best choices within your own caloric needs.

According to the United States Department of Agriculture (USDA), Americans overdo it when it comes to fats and added sugars, consuming—on average—35 percent of their total calories from those sources. The recommendation is to keep the intake of saturated fats and added sugars to only 5 to 15 percent of total calories for most people each day.

▶ EAT BALANCED MEALS

Do you remember the pyramid figure used to represent the food groups and healthy eating patterns? Well, in 2011 that classic pyramid was replaced with MyPlate, a visual representation of the USDA dietary guidelines for general nutrition that serves as a guidance tool to help Americans make their food choices, pointing them in the direction of healthy eating. Key components of MyPlate—and any healthy diet—include variety, balance, and moderation. The amount of food you need daily from each of the food groups really depends on individual characteristics like age, gender, and activity level. In the following sections, I've provided you with the general guidelines for adults. For more detailed information, visit the website at *www.choosemyplate.gov*.

Vegetables

Aim to fill around 30 percent of your plate with vegetables. Make sure to get a variety of vegetables, including those that are green and those that are red- and orange-colored. Don't forget that frozen vegetables will provide you with good nutrients, just like fresh.

Grains

Select whole grains and products made from whole grains. Aim to fill roughly 25 to 30 percent of your plate with grains, which for most adults is about 6 to 8 ounces of grains per day. It is recommended to consume half your daily intake of total grains from whole grains. Look for the words "whole grain" or "100 percent whole grain" on the label and at or near the beginning of the ingredient list. You can also use the Whole Grains Stamp for help determining if you have selected a whole-grain product. A bonus to eating whole grains is that they are packed with fiber, which helps to keep you feeling fuller between meals.

Dairy

Dairy isn't technically located *on* the plate, but that doesn't mean it isn't part of a healthy diet. You can find the milk pictured as a glass next to your plate. Whole milk is not recommended over age two due to the fat content, which also increases the calorie content. The goal is to aim for 3 cups of low-fat or fat-free milk per day, but this can come from yogurt and other low-fat dairy products as well. A key nutrient coming from the dairy group is calcium. But don't worry if you can't tolerate milk due to lactose intolerance or a milk-protein allergy, or if you choose to not drink it because you are vegan; there are other nondairy ways to get your calcium in each day.

Fresh Fruits

Aim to fill around 20 percent of your plate with fruits, and in general always aim to fill half your plate with fruits and vegetables. To help manage your weight, stick with whole fruits and avoid juices, especially those with added sugar.

Protein-Filled Foods

This includes meat, poultry, fish, dry beans, eggs, nuts, and meat substitutes. Aim to fill around 20 percent of your plate with protein-filled foods, focusing on those that are lean and low in fat. Avoid processed meats that have added sodium. Most adults need between 5 and 6 ounces of lean protein each day, but that can vary from person to person. The Recommended Dietary Allowance (RDA) for protein is 0.8 grams per kilogram of body weight. The total needs for the day will include protein grams coming from these protein-filled foods and the protein coming from the other food groups, like dairy and vegetables.

Note that sweets and fats are not a focus on MyPlate, and these are the foods to limit each day. One thing to remember is that there are heart-healthy fats, like those in olive and canola oils, avocado, and nuts, and these are a healthy addition to your diet. Just watch your portions because the calories in fats add up fast—so you don't want to eat too many servings. The fats to cut back on are saturated and trans fatty acids found mainly in cakes, candies, cookies, and other "sweets," as well as those in fried and fast foods.

▶ WHAT'S A SERVING?

This is an area of confusion among many people. It is not uncommon to overestimate your portions when trying to match these up with what really equals one serving. With the increase in portions from restaurants, it is getting harder and harder to tell how much we should be eating at one time. Let's take a look at some basic serving sizes for foods in each of the food groups.

- One serving of grains (1 ounce equivalent): 1 slice of bread; 1 ounce of ready-to-eat cereal; ½ cup of cooked whole-grain cereal, rice, or pasta
- One serving of vegetables (1 cup equivalent): 1 cup of raw leafy greens; 1 cup of other vegetables, cooked or chopped raw; 1 cup of vegetable juice
- One serving of fruit (1 cup equivalent): 1 medium piece of fruit (for example: apple, banana, or orange); 1 cup of chopped, cooked, or canned fruit (look for those canned in water or their own juices); 1 cup fruit juice
- One serving of dairy (1 cup equivalent): 1 cup of milk or yogurt; 1½ ounces of natural cheese; 2 ounces of processed cheese (American); ¼ cup of shredded cheese; ¼ cup of ricotta cheese
- One serving of a protein food (1 ounce equivalent): 1 ounce of cooked lean meat, poultry, or fish; ¼ cup of cooked beans; 1 tablespoon of peanut- or other nut butter; ½ ounce of nuts or seeds; 2 ounces of tofu; 1 egg

It's a good idea to keep these serving sizes in mind because the serving size on the food label of a product is just what that particular food company calls a serving. This may turn out to be more than what is truly considered one serving from the food group according to the guidelines set forth by the USDA, and can result in overeating.

▶ UNDERSTAND CALORIES

While it's important to get the right kind of calories to give your brain what it needs, it is just as important when managing your weight to make sure that those calories are not exceeding what your body needs each day. A calorie is a unit of measurement that relates to the amount of heat released from foods. Everyone has different daily calorie needs, and these can change depending on your activity levels.

These are the general guidelines from the USDA, which are really just a guide or place for you to start before making the adjustments you need to manage your weight, and are determined based on someone who is not physically active: The recommendation for females nineteen to thirty years of age is 1,800–2,000 calories; for males nineteen to thirty years of age, 2,400–2,600 calories; for females thirty-one to fifty years of age, 1,800 calories; for males thirty-one to fifty years of age, 2,200–2,400 calories.

Again, each person's caloric needs will depend on factors like height, weight, age, and activity level. Since the goal is to use tapping to help you lose weight, it's important to remember that your brain can't do *all* the work, and calories do matter when it comes to managing your weight. You should have an idea of the range to aim for each day, and allow yourself to make the right choices to fill those calories each day. One of the common equations used, which accounts for obesity, is the Mifflin–St. Jeor equation. To calculate your own needs, you will need to find your height in centimeters and your weight in kilograms:

Male: BMR = $(10 \times \text{weight}) + (6.25 \times \text{height}) - (5 \times \text{age}) + 5$

Female: BMR = $(10 \times \text{weight}) + (6.25 \times \text{height}) - (5 \times \text{age}) - 161$

Once you have the Basal Metabolic Rate (BMR), you will want to multiply that number by an activity factor:

1.200 = sedentary (little or no exercise)

1.375 = lightly active (light exercise/sports one to three days per week)

1.550 = moderately active (moderate exercise/sports three to five days per week)

1.725 = very active (hard exercise/sports six to seven days per week)

1.900 = extra active (very hard exercise/sports and physical job)

Once you have multiplied the BMR by one of these factors, you have a number that represents the predicted amount of calories you need each day. Of course this is only an estimate, but this is the best place to start. Also, keep in mind this is just a single number, so you may find that some days you are just above this number and other days you are a little below this number. That's to be expected. Remember that your body has the ultimate say as to whether you are eating the right amount of calories. If you notice that you are gaining weight, then your estimated calorie number is too high and you should decrease this because you are really working to lose weight. If you notice that with that number you are maintaining your weight, you will also want to decrease your calorie goals because your plan is to lose weight. It is a little more complex to determine how much to decrease this number by each day, but on average, a decrease of 500 calories will result in around a pound of weight loss per week, so with no changes in your exercise plans, this may be the best number with which to start. If this seems like too much, start with a decrease of 250 calories which will result in a weight loss of ½ pound per week on average.

▶ THE PROBLEM WITH SUGAR

You probably know that too much sugar isn't good for your health, but it does more than just cause weight gain. University of Wisconsin researchers found that the brain may have the same reaction to too many refined added sugars, as it would to a virus or bacteria. This can result in an immune response, which can then lead to cognitive deficits similar to those seen in people with Alzheimer's disease, which can make weight loss difficult. In addition, excessive consumption of refined added sugars can:

- Block cellular membranes, resulting in slower neural communication.
- Increase inflammation in your brain.
- Increase levels of stress hormone cortisol, leading to weight gain or trouble with weight loss.

How can you cut sugar from your diet?

Give Up the Soda

It's no surprise that soda is bad for your health. The empty calories add up quickly, and it doesn't do much to curb your appetite. In addition, glucose, the version of sugar that your body uses for energy, is the main supply of energy utilized by your brain. However, having too much or too little glucose can negatively impact your brain function. Just one soda can provide you with the same amount of glucose as 10 teaspoons of table sugar. That's a lot of sugar coming into your bloodstream at one time considering the normal amount in your bloodstream is equivalent to less than 1 teaspoon of sugar. To compensate for the sudden rush of sugar, your pancreas releases a lot of insulin, all in an effort to bring your blood sugar back into the normal range. Some sugar makes it into your cells, including brain cells, and then the rest will be stored for energy use later (some being stored as fat). About an hour later, your blood sugar, still feeling the effects of all that insulin released, may drop and result in low blood sugar. The constant ups and downs are not only harmful to your health, but can also result in impaired memory and foggy thought patterns.

▶ CUT OUT THE SALT

There is some evidence that having too much sodium can cause a stroke, but there are certainly more factors that play into increasing your risk, including other modifiable factors like obesity and physical activity level. Since high blood pressure is a risk factor for stroke, watching your sodium intake will not only benefit your health in general, but can also lower your risk for stroke—ultimately benefiting your brain.

The previous Dietary Guidelines for Americans called for a daily sodium intake of 2,400 mg. The guidelines now recommend an intake less than 2,300 mg or 1,500 mg per day for people who are more than fifty-one years of age, African Americans (who have an increased risk for high blood pressure), and those who already have high blood pressure, renal failure (chronic), or diabetes. Of course, cutting back on sodium can be beneficial to everyone, especially if you are looking to lose weight, because sodium plays a role in fluid balance in the body. Too much sodium can lead to the body retaining fluid, which in turn leads to a bloated feeling and excess weight to carry around. In order to get rid of some of the excess sodium in your diet, avoid frequent consumption of prepackaged/ prepared meals, cured meats, cheeses, many canned goods, pickles, most soups, soy sauce, and some condiments such as ketchup and mustard. There are other foods like these, so always make sure to check the nutrition facts panel on your foods to see how much sodium a food contains per serving. To cut back on sodium but still enjoy soups and canned vegetables, look for products listed as "low sodium" or "no added salt." You will still want to check the nutrition facts panel for the sodium content, but there is a good chance it will be lower than the "regular" product. You can also cut down your sodium intake by not adding salt to your food at the table and using herbs and spices to flavor foods when cooking at home.

▶ THE MOST IMPORTANT MEAL OF THE DAY

There's a reason why people say breakfast is the most important meal of the day, and although all meals are important and contribute to good health, breakfast really does get you off to the right start. When you wake up in the morning, your body has been in a fasting state overnight. Eating breakfast helps to boost your glucose stores, sending some much-needed fuel to your body—and helping to manage your weight since eating breakfast is linked with weight loss. Of the weight-loss maintainers who provided their weight-loss data to the National Weight Control Registry, 78 percent reported eating breakfast every day. This is one habit that will help you achieve your ideal weight.

Need some breakfast ideas? Try these suggestions or some of the recipes in the following chapter:

- Fortified breakfast cereals (not heavily sweetened) with sliced fruit and fat-free milk
- A whole-grain waffle topped with 1 tablespoon of nut butter and ½ banana
- Two tablespoons of peanut- or almond butter on a whole-wheat bagel

- Cottage cheese and pineapple
- Oatmeal with dried fruits and nuts
- A vegetable-filled egg-white omelet with one slice of whole-grain bread, toasted
- A hard-boiled egg, a piece of fruit, and a slice of whole-grain bread
- Low-fat or nonfat Greek yogurt with fruit

No matter what healthy foods you choose for breakfast, you are taking a step in the right direction by adding this meal into your healthy lifestyle.

TAKE NOTE

Free radicals are unstable atoms with an electron missing, and can roam your body causing damage that has been linked to cancer development and heart disease. Fortunately, antioxidants are substances that stop free radicals from causing damage by stabilizing them. This means that antioxidants are a desirable part of your dietary intake because free radicals can build up in the brain faster than in any other area of your body. In order to benefit from powerful antioxidants like vitamin C or lycopene, follow the MyPlate guidelines and fill half your plate with fruits and vegetables. Aim for dark green vegetables and strive for fall colors (reds, yellows, and oranges). Even purple and blue produce packs an antioxidant punch.

▶ EAT THE RIGHT TYPES OF FATS

Fats play a role in carrying, absorbing, and storing the fat-soluble vitamins (A, D, E, and K). Around 60 percent of your brain is composed of fats, and fat is a component of *all* cell membranes. However, not all fats are created equal—and the type you eat really makes a difference. A diet packed with saturated fats (the bad fats) will not only promote the development of heart disease, but your brain will only be able to make low-quality cell membranes, impacting the ability of neurons to function properly. On the other hand, a diet containing unsaturated fats (the good fats) will help keep your heart healthy and allow your brain cells to produce higher-quality cell membranes, ultimately helping your neurons function at optimal levels. Fat grams pack just over twice the amount of calories found in 1 gram of carbohydrate or protein, and these can add up fast. Unfortunately, it is possible to overdo it, even when you're eating something healthy, so watch how much fat you're eating, and make sure that only around 30 percent of your total daily calories are coming from fats. Good sources of fats include oils (like olive and canola), avocado, nuts, and fatty fish (like salmon and mackerel).

Omega-3 Fatty Acids

As we mentioned before, there are some fats that are good for you, and omega-3 fatty acids fall into this category. Just like other fats, they are calorie dense—but they provide benefits to your health. Currently, research is taking place to see if these essential fatty acids play a role in lowering the risk of dementia and Alzheimer's disease. In addition, a variety of studies have suggested that they may play a factor in weight loss, so make sure they're a staple in your healthy diet. These are some omega-3 fatty acid–containing foods to include in your diet:

- Some fatty, cold-water fish (like salmon, herring, sardines, mackerel, rainbow trout, tuna, and whitefish)
- Canola oil
- Flaxseed oil
- Ground flaxseeds
- Walnuts

Omega-3 fatty acids are great for mental function, including clarity in thoughts, concentration, and the ability to focus, making these a good choice not only for adults but also for children. Unfortunately, the typical American child's diet contains few omega-3 fatty acids, so if you have kids, adding more to your diet may help increase omega-3 intake in your kids' lives, too.

Cut Out Bad Fats

While good fats like omega-3s have positive effects on your brain and help keep you healthy, there is another group of fats that does just the opposite. Unfortunately, the typical American diet is higher in those bad, or unhealthy, fats than in those considered the good fats. These bad fats include saturated fats, which have been linked to heart disease, and are typically found in foods that pack a lot of calories with few vitamins and minerals. Unhealthy fats also include trans fats, which result from a process known as hydrogenation. This technique takes oils and makes them solid, increasing their shelf life, but in the process, the structure of these fats ends up promoting heart disease. You can find both of these kinds of unhealthy fats listed on the nutrition facts panel on packaged foods. These fats are solid—your healthy oils are liquid. Guidelines for saturated fats are to keep your consumption to less than 10 percent of your daily caloric intake. Saturated and trans fats can be found in:

- Many prepackaged, highly processed foods, including commercial baked goods, crackers, chips, and candy.
- Fast foods.
- Fatty cuts of red meat and dark-meat chicken (and the skin).
- Full-fat dairy products, including butter, whole milk, ice cream, and cheese (most margarines, as well, although those are dairy-free).
- Some salad dressings.
- Coconut and palm oils.

Unlike healthy fats, trans fatty acids (you can find them listed on the nutrition facts label and also on the ingredient list as "partially hydrogenated oils") become rigid as a result of the chemical structure, and can get in the way of proper synaptic or electrical nerve cell communication. Because these foods containing trans fats often contain lots of calories (not just from fat—they often have added sugar, too) and very little nutritional benefit, trans fats can thwart your weight-loss efforts. They can also:

- Modify the production of neurotransmitters, such as dopamine.
- Boost LDL (bad) cholesterol levels, while lowering HDL (good) cholesterol levels.
- Increase plaque buildup in blood vessels, which increases the likelihood of blood clots forming, putting both your heart and brain at risk and leading to serious long-term health consequences.
- Interfere with energy production in the mitochondria (the energy factories) of brain cells.
- Raise triglyceride levels in your blood, which may slow down the amount of oxygen circulating throughout your body.

Keeping your diet free (or at least as free as possible) of trans fats benefits you in many ways. You will wind up eliminating many foods from your diet that provide little nutritional benefit, and at the same time you'll keep yourself free from the negative effects that trans fats have on the brain and body.

▶ WATCH YOUR CAFFEINE INTAKE

It may seem like a good idea to get in oodles of caffeine daily, in order to help you stay awake and alert. In fact, you may have even heard that this can help you lose weight. In reality, there is no "miracle cure" here, and too much caffeine can damage your stomach, induce headaches, promote anxiety, and prevent you from getting a good night's sleep. We usually think of coffee right away when thinking about sources of caffeine, but it is important to mention that caffeine is also found in tea leaves and cocoa beans, and in products made from these sources. Other hidden sources that you may not have realized include more than a thousand different over-the-counter and prescription drugs, and even decaffeinated coffee contains a very small amount. When it comes to weight loss, caffeine may boost metabolism for a bit and shed some water weight, but there is not any strong scientific evidence to show that this is dramatic enough to make an impact on your weight long-term, and it certainly does not outweigh the risks associated with excessive consumption of caffeine.

Caffeine Allowance

If your diet contains enough healthy beverages, such as water first and foremost, and perhaps some low-fat or fat-free milk, there is room for you to enjoy some coffee without feeling guilty. The pharmacological active dose for caffeine is listed at 200 milligrams, and the daily recommendation for intake suggests not exceeding the amount in 1 to 3 cups of coffee daily (139 to 417 milligrams). Not sure how much caffeine is found in some common caffeine-containing foods and beverages? Here is a list to help:

- 8 ounces of brewed coffee = 100 milligrams
- 6 ounces of tea brewed from whole leaves = 10–50 milligrams
- 12 ounces of cola = 50 milligrams
- 1 ounce of cocoa (like a milk chocolate bar) = 6 milligrams
- 1 cup of semisweet chocolate chips = 92 milligrams

See, just like with so many things in our lives, moderation plays a key role. Some caffeine can fit easily into a healthy life, and knowing how much is found in the foods and beverages you consume each day will help you make sure you aren't consuming too much.

▶ EAT SUPERFOODS

It may not be the most scientific of terms, but there are some foods that really do deserve to be called *superfoods*, because they provide your body with a lot of the nutrients you need without providing added calories or nutrients you don't need (like artery-clogging fats). In the end, all the foods you eat together impact your weight, but a healthy diet full of a variety of superfoods will help you to lose that extra weight, prevent disease, and live longer. Remember: in addition to tapping, choosing the right foods is an important step to weight loss and will pave the way for you to make healthy lifestyle choices.

Blueberries

Blueberries top the list when it comes to providing your body with protection from disease. Those pretty blue-colored berries are brimming with antioxidant and anti-inflammatory compounds, which have been found in some studies to have the potential to reverse short-term memory loss and slow down the aging process. Research on flavonoids, compounds that are found in blueberries, has been positive so far in showing benefits such as slowing mental decline, and the thought behind this is that flavonoids interact with the proteins found as part of the brain structure, positively impacting the function of the brain and ensuring a healthy body.

While many foods offer up antioxidants, blueberries have a leg up on some of the competition, providing 38 percent more anti-oxidants than red wine. These berries also come out on top when compared with other fruits and vegetables—plus they taste good, which alone should be enough to entice you to add some to your diet. Blueberries are in season (meaning they are generally cheaper at the grocery store) from around late May through the end of summer, but even when they aren't in season you can still enjoy them since they are sold frozen in most grocery stores. Try them in your oatmeal, on a salad, or tossed in Greek yogurt.

But not only blueberries contain flavonoids, so don't pass up other berries and fruits. Flavonoids are antioxidants, and are also found in foods like soybeans, green tea, and cherries. The foods that are most potent when it comes to flavonoids are those boasting red and purple hues. Some other berries not to be missed are goji berries, cranberries, blackberries, mulberries, and boysenberries, all of which are filled with antioxidants and good for your body. Variety is essential to enjoying your healthy diet, so don't forget to change up your berry lineup from time to time.

Whole Grains

Whole grains are a great addition to a healthy diet and provide fiber, which helps in lowering cholesterol and managing weight. But be sure to read the label and ingredient list; if it doesn't say "whole grain," you aren't getting the full benefits. Additionally, a food may have whole grains but could be mixed with refined grains—so look for "100 percent whole grain" on the label and check to make sure the first ingredient listed is whole grain. Oats and wheat are great whole grains to start with and are easy to find. Other great whole grains include barley, corn, millet, rice, buckwheat, bulgur, farro, spelt, and rye. Aim to make half your grain intake each day from 100 percent whole-grain foods. This works out to about three to five servings per day (as a general goal).

A serving is ½ cup cooked brown rice, ½ cup cooked oatmeal, 1 slice of 100 percent whole-grain bread, 1 ounce of uncooked whole-grain pasta, or 1 cup of 100 percent whole-grain cereal. Or, consider it this way: 16 grams of whole-grain ingredients counts as one serving of whole grains. Look for the Whole Grain Stamp on foods to make it easy to see how much you are eating. Aim to eat at least three foods with the 100 percent Whole Grain Stamp or six foods with any Whole Grain Stamp to help meet your goals. For more information on whole grains, check out *www.wholegrains council.org.*

Fish

Fish is often touted as a superfood, and with good reason. Many fish are filled with omega-3 fatty acids. When coupled with nutrients like protein, vitamins, and minerals, they work hard to keep you healthy. The American Heart Association recommends eating two 3½-ounce servings of fish weekly, particularly in the form of fatty fish. Of course, there is some concern when it comes to fish and seafood—some are high in mercury, a harmful toxin. When it comes to eating fish, the best practice is to eat enough to receive a benefit from the positive aspects of fish, but not so much as to consume too many environmental pollutants that can be found in fish. Watch your intake of species that are higher in mercury, including shark, king mackerel, swordfish, and tilefish. The fish highest in omega-3 content include albacore tuna, sardines, salmon, mackerel, lake trout, and herring. The five most commonly eaten fish that are low in mercury are shrimp, canned light tuna, salmon, polluck, and catfish. A good rule of thumb is to eat a variety of fish to minimize any potentially adverse effects due to environmental pollutants.

For weight loss, make sure you are including fish as a healthy part of your diet. The preparation of these foods will make a difference as well, so aim for grilling, broiling, poaching, or baking, rather than frying your fish. Look for low-sodium marinades, sauces, and seasonings or cook your fish in a little olive oil and lemon juice. For a healthy meal, enjoy your fish with some vegetables and a whole grain.

> **TAKE NOTE**
>
> There is no denying that salmon is a superior choice when it comes to eating fish. However, not all salmon are raised equal. Your best bet, when it comes to getting those omega-3s without the possibility of antibiotics and with fewer environmental toxins, is wild salmon. Most of the time Atlantic salmon will be farmed, so look for Pacific kinds and check to see if it is wild. Just remember that this can get pricey, so it doesn't need to be the only fish in your diet. Remember to aim for variety when it comes to fish and omega-3s. Looking to cut down on costs? Try canned varieties of wild salmon.

Avocado

There are many good-for-you green foods out there, but the superfood that often gets overlooked is avocado, which contains heart-healthy fats. The potassium content in avocado helps to lower blood pressure, and when coupled with this food's tendency to increase blood flow, avocados truly are a benefit to your brain. Since this is a fatty food, it helps you to better absorb fat-soluble vitamins like A, D, E, and K. Avocados also have anti-inflammatory properties. But, as with so many foods, portion size does matter. Since this is a fat-containing food, the calories can add up quickly, so watch how much you are eating; you can still get the health benefits without overdoing it. In one-fifth of a medium avocado, which is about 1 ounce, there are roughly 60 calories, 6 grams of fat (5 grams of which are unsaturated and heart-healthy), and 3 grams of fiber. Not sure what to do with an avocado, other than make guacamole? Try it as a topping on a sandwich or salad.

Nuts

Just like avocados, nuts are a good source of healthy fats and also supply your body with vitamins, minerals, fiber, and protein. As a bonus, nuts also provide the resources your body needs for your brain to produce mood-boosting serotonin, which can help you get in a positive mood for tapping. At the top of the list for keeping your heart healthy and your blood flowing are walnuts, pecans, almonds, and hazelnuts.

All nuts are high in calories per serving because they are filled with good fats, so limit your intake to 1 ounce (roughly twenty-four almonds) daily in order to keep your weight-loss goals on track. Don't forget to aim for unsalted nuts. A 1-ounce serving of almonds contains around 160 calories, 14 grams of fat, 3 grams of fiber, and 6 grams of protein. No need to get stuck on one nut. Try a variety that includes pistachios, walnuts, almonds, pecans, cashews, hazelnuts, and Brazil nuts.

Quinoa

This Incan grainlike food, integral to agriculture in the Andes region of South America, is currently gaining popularity in North America—and for good reason. Very few plant foods contain all of the essential amino acids, which are typically found only in animal protein sources. Quinoa (pronounced in the United States as *keen-wa*, although overseas it's pronounced *key-no-ah*), along with soy, does contain all essential amino acids, making it a complete protein. Quinoa is also packed with fiber, manganese, copper, folate, magnesium, and other nutrients and is low in fat, which makes it a wise addition to any meal. One of those essential amino acids (meaning that it must come from the diet, since the body can't make it) is lysine, essential for tissue growth and repair.

When it comes to your waistline, keep the portion size in mind. A full cup of cooked quinoa provides around 220 calories, 4 grams of fat, 39 grams of carbohydrates, 5 grams of fiber, and 8 grams of protein. It makes a nice side dish for fish (or any lean meat), and is also great served at breakfast topped with berries. Quinoa can be found in many mainstream grocery stores these days, so if you have trouble locating it, don't be shy—ask someone to help you.

Soy

There are many benefits to including soy as part of your diet. It is low in fat and a great source of protein. Soy has been linked with lowering blood cholesterol levels as well as reducing blood clots, resulting in better cardiovascular health. Soy also enhances the elasticity of arterial walls, allowing for better blood flow. The biggest benefit of eating soy is that it's a low-fat source of complete protein, which is beneficial to health when it is used to replace saturated fats from animal sources of protein. Sources of soy include tofu, edamame (immature, green soybeans), soymilk, mature soybeans, tempeh (fermented soybean cake), and soy-based "dairy" products. You can also find soy in soy sauce and miso (fermented soy paste), but watch out for the sodium content. Soybean oil is another source—but, like all oils, too much can negatively impact weight, so pay attention to portion size.

▶ EAT CHOCOLATE IN MODERATION

Part of eating a balanced diet is treating yourself, in moderation. Fortunately, chocolate is good for your body, but only when it's eaten in moderation. Henriette van Praag and colleagues from the Salk Institute found that a compound in cocoa, known as epicatechin, combined with exercise, promoted functional changes in an area of the brain that plays a role in learning and memory. There is room in a healthy diet for a little chocolate, and fitting some in here and there will help you avoid feeling deprived or like you have to hide from a chocolate craving. A 1-ounce square, up to three times a week, is enough to get the benefits for your brain, and also benefits your sweet tooth. The benefit is in the cocoa itself, so stick with dark or even semisweet chocolate. Milk chocolate is not the best choice because it has added ingredients and saturated fat that reduces the benefits that chocolate can provide. Chocolate's benefits include the following:

- It contains tryptophan, the precursor required to make the neurotransmitter serotonin, which boosts your mood and makes you happy. No wonder we crave it when we're feeling down!
- It contains flavonoids that act as antioxidants and help protect your cells.
- It's a good source of magnesium, which is essential for many reactions involved in metabolism. It helps the body more efficiently metabolize your food into energy.
- It contains phytochemicals, which help prevent arterial damage.

In addition, chocolate contains theobromine, caffeine, and other substances that just might boost your concentration and help you find the focus you need to create healthy meals and guide your body to its best shape yet.

CHAPTER 7

THE RECIPES

The first place to start for a healthy brain and body is tapping, but establishing a healthy, appropriate diet is also an important part of the weight-loss journey. A poor diet will not only promote weight issues and malnutrition, but will also prevent you from thinking clearly and making wise decisions. When it comes to getting yourself to the weight you desire, you need to pay attention to what, and how much, you are eating. The delicious recipes found in this chapter will help you, so use them to guide your weight-loss plan.

Getting the right balance of nutrients will help you manage your weight and help your body function at its best, but it's up to you to use tapping to help resolve the emotional issues that make losing weight difficult, make the right choices, incorporate these healthy foods, and fill the rest of your diet with nutrient-rich choices that will keep you feeling satisfied, knowing that you are feeding your body the right way.

BREAKFAST AND BRUNCH

APPETIZERS AND DIPS

SOUPS AND SALADS

▶ BREAKFAST AND BRUNCH

BAKED SCRAMBLED EGGS

YIELDS 12 SERVINGS

½ cup butter

20 eggs

2 teaspoons salt

1¾ cups fat-free milk

½ cup shredded low-fat cheese

1. Preheat oven to 350°F.
2. In a glass measuring cup, heat the butter in the microwave until melted.
3. In a separate medium bowl whisk the eggs, salt, and milk.
4. Pour the melted butter and then the eggs into a 9" × 13" baking dish.
5. Bake uncovered for 8 minutes, then stir and add cheese if desired. Bake for 10 to 15 more minutes or until eggs are set.

PER SERVING: CALORIES: 212 | FAT: 16G | PROTEIN: 13G | SODIUM: 561MG | FIBER: 0G | CARBOHYDRATES: 2G | SUGAR: 2G

TAKE NOTE

Eggs provide a tremendous amount of protein and very few carbohydrates, and they make you feel full. You should have one egg a day, but remember that so many things we consume daily already contain eggs. Before you have your daily dose of egg, make sure your other meals and snacks do not contain eggs, or you could overdo it.

LOW-FAT EGG AND SPINACH CUPCAKES
YIELDS 5 SERVINGS

10 ounces chopped frozen spinach

2 eggs

1 cup skim ricotta cheese

1 cup low-fat shredded mozzarella cheese

1. Preheat oven to 350°F.
2. Place cupcake liners in 12-hole cupcake tin.
3. Heat spinach in microwave until soft and warm.
4. Whip the eggs in a medium bowl and add the spinach. Blend together.
5. Fold in the ricotta and shredded cheese.
6. Fill each cup with egg-spinach mixture, about ½" per cup.
7. Bake 30–35 minutes.

PER SERVING: CALORIES: 142 | FAT: 6G | PROTEIN: 17G | SODIUM: 345MG | FIBER: 2G | CARBOHYDRATES: 5G | SUGAR: 1G

EGG AND CHEESE BREAKFAST PIZZA

YIELDS 8 SERVINGS

1 tablespoon all-purpose flour

1 (16-ounce) frozen pizza dough

Cooking spray

1½ cups Egg Beaters

½ cup fat-free milk

½ cup low-fat cheese, any flavor

1. Preheat oven to 375°F.
2. Sprinkle flour on a flat surface and roll out the pizza dough into a 12" circle, building up the edges so they're thick and high. Place the dough on a nonstick baking sheet and then prick the dough thoroughly with a fork.
3. Bake until light brown, about 15 minutes.
4. While the crust is baking, coat a skillet with cooking spray and beat the Egg Beaters and milk in a large bowl.
5. Scramble the mixture over medium heat, then place scrambled eggs on pizza crust and sprinkle with cheese.
6. Bake 7 minutes to melt the cheese, then slice with knife or pizza roller.

PER SERVING: CALORIES: 170 | FAT: 3G | PROTEIN: 11G | SODIUM: 500MG | FIBER: 1G | CARBOHYDRATES: 26G | SUGAR: 5G

EGGS BENEDICT
YIELDS 4 SERVINGS

3 tablespoons skim milk

½ cup low-fat mayonnaise

4 eggs

4 slices bacon

4 slices whole-wheat bread, or 2 whole-wheat English muffins

1. Mix the skim milk with the mayonnaise and heat in the microwave for about 40 seconds to warm.
2. Crack each egg into individual microwavable bowls, being careful not to break the yolks.
3. Cover each bowl with plastic wrap and microwave on high until the whites are cooked and yolks firm, about 2 minutes.
4. In a skillet, cook the bacon.
5. Place the bacon on the whole-wheat bread slices.
6. Add the eggs on the bacon and top each egg with 2 tablespoons of mayonnaise mixture.

PER SERVING: CALORIES: 216 | FAT: 12G | PROTEIN: 12G | SODIUM: 593MG | FIBER: 2G | CARBOHYDRATES: 15G | SUGAR: 3G

STUFFED FRENCH TOAST
YIELDS 4 SERVINGS

Butter-flavored cooking spray

4 slices French bread

4 teaspoons reduced-fat cream cheese

4 teaspoons favorite preserves

1 cup skim milk

1 teaspoon vanilla

1 teaspoon cinnamon, or to taste

½ teaspoon nutmeg, or to taste

1. Prepare a skillet with the butter-flavored spray.
2. Slice French bread into 1"-thick slices.
3. Cut a pocket through the top of each slice, ¾ of the way through the bread.
4. Insert 1 teaspoon of cream cheese and 1 teaspoon of preserves into each slice.
5. Combine milk, vanilla, cinnamon, and nutmeg in a shallow bowl to make the batter.
6. Dip the bread in the batter and cook in the skillet until golden and slightly firm.

PER SERVING: CALORIES: 238 | FAT: 2G | PROTEIN: 10G | SODIUM: 380MG | FIBER: 2G | CARBOHYDRATES: 45G | SUGAR: 8G

TAKE NOTE
The fresher your bread, the more it falls apart in the batter. Use bread that is nearing the end of its shelf life. It will be a little tougher and will hold together better when soaked in batter.

OATMEAL BANANA BREAD

YIELDS 20 SERVINGS

Light cooking spray

1½ cups flour

⅔ cup sugar

1½ teaspoons baking powder

¼ teaspoon baking soda

¼ teaspoon salt

¾ cup dry oatmeal

1 cup mashed bananas

½ cup soymilk

¼ cup walnut oil

1 teaspoon vanilla extract

2 eggs

1. Preheat oven to 350°F.
2. Spray an 8" × 4" loaf pan with light cooking spray.
3. Mix all dry ingredients in a large bowl.
4. Mix the mashed banana, soymilk, oil, vanilla, and eggs in a small bowl.
5. Blend the wet ingredients in with the dry ingredients.
6. Spoon batter into the prepared pan and bake for 50 minutes, or until light golden brown on top.
7. Cool on a wire rack for 20 minutes.
8. Remove the bread from the pan and cool thoroughly on the rack before serving.

PER SERVING: CALORIES: 116 | FAT: 4G | PROTEIN: 2G | SODIUM: 92MG | FIBER: 1G | CARBOHYDRATES: 19G | SUGAR: 8G

CHERRY–BERRY SCONES

YIELDS 8 SERVINGS

2½ cups all-purpose flour	2 whole eggs, beaten
2½ teaspoons baking powder	⅔ cup skim milk
1 tablespoon sugar	½ cup frozen cherries, thawed
1 teaspoon salt	½ cup frozen blueberries, thawed
4 tablespoons unsalted butter	4 egg whites

1. Preheat oven to 450°F.
2. Combine flour, baking powder, sugar, and salt in a large bowl. Cut the butter into small bits and mix with the flour until mixture is crumbly.
3. Add whole eggs, milk, and fruit and mix until blended well.
4. Sprinkle extra flour over a clean, flat work space and knead the dough into an 8" circle. Cut the circle into eight wedges and transfer to a nonstick baking sheet. Brush top of scone wedges with the egg whites.
5. Bake 15–20 minutes or until scones turn golden.

PER SERVING: CALORIES: 243 | FAT: 7G | PROTEIN: 8G | SODIUM: 552MG | FIBER: 1G | CARBOHYDRATES: 35G | SUGAR: 5G

TAKE NOTE

Scones are traditionally served with preserves and clotted cream, but serve these delicious scones with jam or honey to save on calories. They are popular teatime snacks, but they also work well for breakfast.

BLUEBERRY MUFFINS
YIELDS 12 SERVINGS

Light cooking spray	½ teaspoon salt
2 cups flour	1 cup low-fat buttermilk
½ cup sugar	1 egg
1 teaspoon baking powder	½ cup butter, softened
½ teaspoon baking soda	1 cup blueberries

1. Preheat oven to 400°F. Prepare a muffin tin with light cooking spray.
2. Mix the flour, sugar, baking powder, baking soda, and salt in a medium bowl.
3. Whisk buttermilk and egg together. Then add the butter and beat well. Add to flour mixture. Fold in the blueberries.
4. Spoon batter into 12 muffin cups and bake for 20 minutes, or until the muffins spring back when touched.

PER SERVING: CALORIES: 197 | FAT: 8G | PROTEIN: 4G | SODIUM: 220MG | FIBER: 1G | CARBOHYDRATES: 27G | SUGAR: 11G

TAKE NOTE

A great way to make sure all of your muffins are the exact same size is to use an ice cream scoop to spoon the batter into the tins. For high-rising, rounded tops on muffins, preheat your oven to 500°F. As soon as you put the muffins into the oven, decrease the temperature to 400°F and keep an eye on the muffins because the baking time will go down.

TRIPLE-PLAY CHOCOLATE-BANANA NUT MUFFINS
YIELDS 20 SERVINGS

1 cup boiling water

2 cups wheat bran

1 cup oat bran

½ cup applesauce

1 cup honey

2 egg whites

2 cups skim milk

2 cups flour

3 teaspoons baking soda

½ teaspoon salt

½ cup chopped walnuts

1 cup mashed banana

½ cup semisweet chocolate chips

1. Preheat oven to 400°F.
2. Mix boiling water and bran and let stand until water is mostly absorbed.
3. Cream applesauce and honey. Add egg whites and milk, then add the bran.
4. Add the flour, soda, and salt. Fold in nuts, mashed bananas, and chocolate chips.
5. Pour an equal amount of batter into each cup of a mini–muffin tin. Bake for 20 minutes or until toothpick inserted into the muffins comes out clean.

PER SERVING: CALORIES: 195 | FAT: 4G | PROTEIN: 5G | SODIUM: 265MG | FIBER: 4G | CARBOHYDRATES: 39G | SUGAR: 20G

RAISIN MUFFINS
YIELDS 6 SERVINGS

2 cups dry oat bran

¼ cup brown sugar

1 tablespoon baking powder

2 egg whites

1 cup low-fat buttermilk

½ cup molasses

½ cup unsweetened applesauce

¾ cup raisins

1. Preheat oven to 450°F.
2. Mix the oat bran, brown sugar, and baking powder in a large bowl.
3. Beat egg whites until foamy in a small bowl. Stir in buttermilk and molasses.
4. Add the buttermilk mixture to the oat bran mixture, then fold in the applesauce and raisins.
5. Pour an equal amount of batter into each cup of a muffin tin. Bake until tops are golden, about 20 minutes.

PER SERVING: CALORIES: 245 | FAT: 3G | PROTEIN: 9G | SODIUM: 319MG | FIBER: 6G | CARBOHYDRATES: 61G | SUGAR: 36G

▶ APPETIZERS AND DIPS

CHICKEN "WINGS"
YIELDS 10 SERVINGS

2 pounds chicken tenders	1 teaspoon salt
⅓ cup soy sauce	1 teaspoon hot sauce
¼ cup apple cider vinegar	4 cloves garlic, minced
2 tablespoons Dijon mustard	½ cup minced onion
¼ cup honey	1 cup low-fat sour cream
¼ cup brown sugar	2 cups celery sticks

1. Cut chicken tenders in half crosswise. In heavy-duty food-storage bag, combine remaining ingredients except sour cream and celery; mix well. Add chicken tenders and seal bag. Place bag in baking dish; refrigerate for at least 8 hours, up to 24 hours.
2. When ready to prepare, preheat oven to 400°F. Drain chicken tenders, reserving marinade. Arrange tenders in single layer in large pan. Drizzle with ½ cup of the reserved marinade. Bake for 20–25 minutes or until chicken is thoroughly cooked.
3. Meanwhile, place remaining marinade in small saucepan. Bring to a simmer over high heat, then reduce heat to low and cook for 10–15 minutes, stirring frequently, until mixture is syrupy. Combine with sour cream and serve as a dipping sauce for chicken along with celery.

PER SERVING: CALORIES: 340 | FAT: 17G | PROTEIN: 16G | SODIUM: 1297MG | FIBER: 2G | CARBOHYDRATES: 30G | SUGAR: 15G

SPINACH PUFFS
YIELDS 4 SERVINGS

¾ cup chopped mushrooms, including stems

¼ cup canola oil

1 (5-ounce) package frozen chopped spinach, thawed, water squeezed out

¾ cup shredded Gruyère cheese

2 thawed puff pastry sheets

¼ cup low-cholesterol margarine, melted

1. Sauté mushrooms in canola oil in a skillet over medium heat until mushrooms begin to soften.
2. Add spinach and cheese to mushrooms and stir. Once cheese is melted, remove from heat.
3. Place one pastry sheet on a cookie sheet and brush with half of the melted margarine.
4. Spread half of spinach mixture on prepared pastry sheet.
5. Cover with the remaining pastry sheet and brush with remaining melted margarine.
6. Top with remaining spinach.
7. Cover and refrigerate for at least an hour.
8. Preheat oven to temperature recommend on puff pastry package or 400°F. Cut into four 1" wheels, like a pizza slice.
9. Bake for 15 minutes or until brown.

PER SERVING: CALORIES: 447 | FAT: 41G | PROTEIN: 9G | SODIUM: 182MG | FIBER: 2G | CARBOHYDRATES: 12G | SUGAR: 1G

WHITE BEAN BRUSCHETTA

YIELDS 6 SERVINGS

1 (15-ounce) can cannellini beans, rinsed and drained

⅓ teaspoon thyme

¼ teaspoon seasoned salt

Ground pepper, to taste

2 tablespoons chopped Vidalia onion

1 small clove garlic, crushed

⅓ cup low-cholesterol margarine, melted

1 loaf Italian bread, cut into 12 (1") slices

1. Put beans, thyme, salt, pepper, onions, and garlic in a blender or food processor. Purée until smooth.
2. Lightly spread margarine on bread.
3. Spread bean paste on each slice of bread.
4. Place slices of bread under broiler for 1 minute, or serve cold.

PER SERVING: CALORIES: 337 | FAT: 13G | PROTEIN: 11G | SODIUM: 470MG | FIBER: 5G | CARBOHYDRATES: 46G | SUGAR: 1G

HONEY AND CHEESE-STUFFED FIGS
YIELDS 4 SERVINGS

8 medium ripe figs

⅓ cup crumbled Gorgonzola cheese

1 teaspoon olive oil

¼ cup honey

1. Preheat oven to 300°F.
2. Wash and dry figs. Make a slit in each one from top to bottom.
3. Stuff each fig with the cheese.
4. Roll each fig in olive oil and shake excess off.
5. Place figs on baking sheet and bake, watching them until they plump up, about 30 minutes.
6. Drizzle honey on baked figs when ready to serve.

PER SERVING: CALORIES: 188 | FAT: 5G | PROTEIN: 3G | SODIUM: 159MG | FIBER: 3G | CARBOHYDRATES: 37G | SUGAR: 34G

CHEESE STRAWS

YIELDS 6 SERVINGS

1 (15-ounce) package pie crust mix

½ cup shredded low-fat cheddar cheese

½ teaspoon cayenne pepper

Light cooking spray

1. Preheat oven to 350°F.
2. Prepare pie crust mix according to directions.
3. Sprinkle shredded cheese over pie crust dough, then work it into the dough with your hands.
4. Roll dough into a circle, about 8" around, ⅓" thick.
5. Cut long strips about 1" wide.
6. Sprinkle both sides of each strip with cayenne pepper.
7. Place strips on baking sheet, lightly sprayed with cooking spray.
8. Bake until slightly brown.

PER SERVING: CALORIES: 394 | FAT: 24G | PROTEIN: 7G | SODIUM: 603MG | FIBER: OG | CARBOHYDRATES: 39G | SUGAR: OG

MARINARA DIP
YIELDS 4 SERVINGS

1 (8-ounce) can diced tomatoes

2 cloves garlic, crushed

1 teaspoon red pepper flakes

1 tablespoon parsley flakes

¼ teaspoon lemon juice

½ tablespoon anchovy paste

½ tablespoon extra-virgin olive oil

Salt and pepper, to taste

1. Heat all ingredients in a medium saucepan and cook over low heat for about 5 minutes, or until well blended.
2. Add salt and pepper to taste.
3. Remove from heat, place in a bowl, and serve with baked chips or vegetables.

PER SERVING: CALORIES: 42 | FAT: 2G | PROTEIN: 1G | SODIUM: 219MG | FIBER: 1G | CARBOHYDRATES: 5G | SUGAR: 3G

TAKE NOTE
Marinara sauce originated in Naples, Italy as a meatless sauce used on sailing ships. The lack of meat, sheer simplicity, and high acid content of this sauce means that it does not easily spoil and therefore will keep in the refrigerator for weeks.

GINGERBREAD FRUIT DIP

YIELDS 12 SERVINGS

1 (8-ounce) package cream cheese, softened

½ cup low-fat sour cream

⅓ cup brown sugar

¼ cup maple syrup or light molasses

2 tablespoons chopped candied ginger

½ teaspoon ground ginger

½ teaspoon cinnamon

¼ teaspoon nutmeg

1. In medium bowl, beat cream cheese until light and fluffy. Gradually add sour cream, beating until smooth.
2. Add sugar and beat well. Gradually add molasses and beat until smooth. Stir in remaining ingredients.
3. Cover and chill for at least 3 hours before serving with fresh fruit.

PER SERVING: CALORIES: 130 | FAT: 8G | PROTEIN: 2G | SODIUM: 71MG | FIBER: 0G | CARBOHYDRATES: 14G | SUGAR: 11G

TAKE NOTE

Candied ginger is also known as crystallized ginger. It is made of pieces of ginger root simmered in a sugar syrup, then rolled in sugar. You can make your own by combining ¾ cup sugar with ¾ cup water and bringing it to a simmer. Add ½ cup peeled and chopped fresh ginger root; simmer for 25 minutes. Drain, dry, then roll in sugar to coat.

SMOKED SALMON DIP

YIELDS 4 SERVINGS

1 cup plain nonfat yogurt

2 large seedless cucumbers, peeled and finely chopped

1 tablespoon dill

1 teaspoon lemon juice

1 teaspoon virgin olive oil

¼ pound smoked salmon

Salt and pepper, to taste

1. Mix all ingredients except the salmon, salt, and pepper until well blended.
2. Chop salmon into small pieces and mix into other ingredients.
3. Add salt and pepper to taste.
4. Refrigerate for at least 1 hour, then serve with baked chips or vegetables.

PER SERVING: CALORIES: 129 | FAT: 2G | PROTEIN: 9G | SODIUM: 325MG | FIBER: OG | CARBOHYDRATES: 18G | SUGAR: 8G

ARTICHOKE SPINACH DIP

YIELDS 4 SERVINGS

Light cooking spray

2 cloves garlic, minced

1 tablespoon olive oil

1½ cups part-skim ricotta cheese

½ teaspoon thyme

1 teaspoon lemon zest

½ teaspoon cayenne pepper

1 (9-ounce) box frozen artichokes, thawed and drained

8 ounces frozen spinach, thawed and drained

¼ cup grated Parmesan cheese

¼ cup bread crumbs

Salt and pepper to taste

1. Preheat oven to 350°F. Prepare a baking dish with light cooking spray.
2. In a skillet, sauté the garlic in olive oil until garlic begins to soften.
3. Pulse ricotta cheese, thyme, lemon zest, and cayenne pepper in food processor until creamy.
4. Add artichokes, spinach, and Parmesan cheese; pulse again, but keep it chunky.
5. Transfer artichoke mixture into baking dish sprayed with light cooking spray.
6. Sprinkle bread crumbs and garlic over artichoke mixture. Season with salt and pepper.
7. Bake for 20 minutes or until warmed through.
8. Serve with chips or vegetables.

PER SERVING: CALORIES: 246 | FAT: 13G | PROTEIN: 17G | SODIUM: 338MG | FIBER: 5G | CARBOHYDRATES: 18G | SUGAR: 1G

HOT CRAB DIP
YIELDS 6 SERVINGS

1 pound crabmeat

2 scallions, finely chopped

4 ounces fat-free cream cheese, softened

½ cup light mayonnaise

¼ cup grated Parmesan cheese

⅓ teaspoon horseradish

Salt, to taste

1. Mix all ingredients in medium bowl.
2. Heat in microwave for 1–2 minutes, until hot.
3. Serve with baked chips or vegetables.

PER SERVING: CALORIES: 140 | FAT: 7G | PROTEIN: 15G | SODIUM: 747MG | FIBER: 0G | CARBOHYDRATES: 4G | SUGAR: 2G

▶ SOUPS AND SALADS

WHITE BEAN SOUP
YIELDS 4 SERVINGS

½ pound dried white beans

¼ cup olive oil

5 garlic cloves, crushed

2 carrots, peeled and chopped

2 celery stalks, chopped

16 ounces low-sodium chicken broth

6 cups water

1 bay leaf

¼ cup chopped parsley

1. Cover the beans in a bowl of water and soak overnight in the refrigerator.
2. Drain the beans and place them in a large pot.
3. Add the olive oil, garlic, carrots, celery, chicken broth, and water and bring everything to a boil. Cook covered for 15 minutes.
4. Reduce heat to a simmer; add the bay leaf and parsley.
5. Continue to simmer until beans are tender, about 2 hours, then remove bay leaf and serve.

PER SERVING: CALORIES: 350 | FAT: 15G | PROTEIN: 16G | SODIUM: 83MG | FIBER: 10G | CARBOHYDRATES: 41G | SUGAR: 3G

FRENCH ONION SOUP
YIELDS 8 SERVINGS

2 large white onions, thinly sliced

2 tablespoons margarine

32 ounces low-sodium beef broth

2 tablespoons Worcestershire sauce

1 teaspoon freshly ground pepper

8 medium slices French bread, toasted

¾ cup nonfat grated cheese, any type

1. Preheat broiler.
2. In a large pot, cook the onions with the margarine over medium heat until brown. Add the broth, Worcestershire sauce, and pepper; bring to a boil.
3. Pour into 8 individual ovenproof bowls. Top with toasted bread and grated cheese. Place under broiler, heat until cheese bubbles, and serve.

PER SERVING: CALORIES: 319 | FAT: 5G | PROTEIN: 18G | SODIUM: 894MG | FIBER: 3G | CARBOHYDRATES: 50G | SUGAR: 5G

TAKE NOTE
History tells us that French onion soup was created by King Louis XV of France. He wanted something to eat late one night but only had onions, butter, and champagne, so he mixed them together and the first French onion soup was born.

BLACK BEAN SOUP

YIELDS 4 SERVINGS

1 (15-ounce) can black beans, rinsed and drained, divided

¼ cup mild salsa

2 cups water

1 cup chopped tomatoes

1 teaspoon ground cumin

1 teaspoon sugar

1. Set aside 4 tablespoons of black beans to use later. Place remaining beans, salsa, water, and tomato chunks in a large pot and mix. Mix in the cumin and sugar.
2. Place all ingredients in a blender and purée until smooth. Place back into a large pot and heat on medium until bubbling. Serve hot and garnish with the reserved black beans.

PER SERVING: CALORIES: 116 | FAT: 1G | PROTEIN: 7G | SODIUM: 526MG | FIBER: 8G | CARBOHYDRATES: 22G | SUGAR: 3G

TAKE NOTE

Black beans help lower cholesterol and are high in fiber, which helps slow rising blood sugar levels. Black beans are a particularly wise choice for people with diabetes or hypoglycemia. They are a virtually fat-free protein as well.

BEEF CHILI
YIELDS 4 SERVINGS

3 cloves garlic, minced

1 tablespoon canola oil

1 pound lean ground beef

1 (15-ounce) can diced tomatoes

1 (16-ounce) can red kidney beans

½ teaspoon cumin seed

½ teaspoon oregano

1½ tablespoons chili powder

Salt and pepper, to taste

1. Sauté garlic in the canola oil in a heavy skillet over medium heat until fragrant, about 1 minute.
2. Add the ground beef, mixing thoroughly until meat is brown.
3. Reduce heat to low. Add the tomatoes and beans, mixing thoroughly.
4. Add the cumin, oregano, chili powder, salt, and pepper.
5. Cover and simmer for 1 hour, stirring occasionally. Serve immediately.

PER SERVING: CALORIES: 309 | FAT: 10G | PROTEIN: 32G | SODIUM: 609MG | FIBER: 8G | CARBOHYDRATES: 23G | SUGAR: 5G

GAZPACHO

YIELDS 8 SERVINGS

6 tomatoes, peeled and chopped

1 purple onion, finely chopped

1 seedless cucumber, chopped and peeled

1 green pepper, seeded and chopped

2 celery stalks, chopped

3 tablespoons chopped parsley

2 tablespoons chopped chives

1 clove garlic, crushed

¼ cup olive oil

3 tablespoons lemon juice

1 teaspoon sugar

Salt and pepper, to taste

4 cups tomato juice

1. Mix all ingredients in a large pot. Combine thoroughly.
2. Transfer to a blender and blend in portions.
3. Refrigerate in bowls for 2–3 hours to chill before serving.

PER SERVING: CALORIES: 120 | FAT: 7G | PROTEIN: 2G | SODIUM: 355MG | FIBER: 3G | CARBOHYDRATES: 13G | SUGAR: 8G

TAKE NOTE

Gazpacho is a cold Spanish soup, created for the summer to cool off during the hot, humid weather. It's traditionally made with tomatoes and served with hard-boiled eggs.

CUCUMBER AND RED ONION SALAD
YIELDS 4 SERVINGS

2 large cucumbers

2 cups salted water

1 large red onion, sliced into thin rings

¼ cup apple cider vinegar

½ cup canola oil

Salt and pepper, to taste

1 teaspoon sugar

1. Peel cucumbers, halve them, and scoop out the seeds.
2. Slice cucumber and place in a bowl with salted water for 20 minutes.
3. Drain cucumber slices.
4. Combine cucumber slices and onion slices.
5. Add the rest of the ingredients, mix well, and refrigerate until ready to serve.

PER SERVING: CALORIES: 280 | FAT: 28G | PROTEIN: 1G | SODIUM: 5MG | FIBER: 2G | CARBOHYDRATES: 8G | SUGAR: 5G

PEAR AND WATERCRESS SALAD

YIELDS 4 SERVINGS

2 pears

3 tablespoons canola oil, divided

1½ tablespoons apple cider vinegar

Salt and pepper, to taste

1 teaspoon whole-grain mustard

½ cup watercress, washed, dried, stems trimmed

1 cup arugula, washed, dried, stems trimmed

2 ounces bleu cheese, crumbled

1. Core the pears. Cut into ¾" slices.
2. In 1 teaspoon of canola oil, sauté the pears over medium heat until brown. Remove from heat and set aside.
3. Mix the remaining oil with the vinegar, salt, and pepper.
4. Add mustard, whisking until dressing is slightly thick.
5. Mix watercress and arugula in a plastic bag.
6. Put into salad bowl; add bleu cheese.
7. Add pears to salad bowl. Top with dressing. Serve immediately.

PER SERVING: CALORIES: 196 | FAT: 14G | PROTEIN: 4G | SODIUM: 219MG | FIBER: 3G | CARBOHYDRATES: 14G | SUGAR: 9G

CRISPY COBB SALAD
YIELDS 4 SERVINGS

4 ounces arugula

2 cups shredded white-meat chicken, boiled

1 large tomato, chopped

2 hard-boiled eggs, finely chopped

1 ripe avocado, pitted and sliced into small pieces

3 slices cooked bacon, crumbled

½ cup bottled low-calorie bleu cheese dressing

1. Layer shallow salad bowl as follows: arugula, chicken, tomato, eggs, avocado, and bacon.
2. Cover with blue cheese dressing and serve immediately.

PER SERVING: CALORIES: 310 | FAT: 17G | PROTEIN: 30G | SODIUM: 528MG | FIBER: 4G | CARBOHYDRATES: 11G | SUGAR: 3G

TAKE NOTE

Layering is a fun and different way to serve a salad, with a surprise as you dig in. It also provides a nicer, more ordered presentation, and it's easy to prepare since you don't have to fuss over mixing the salad perfectly.

ASIAN BEEF SALAD

YIELDS 4 SERVINGS

¾ pound flank steak, thinly sliced and rolled in black pepper

3 tablespoons lime juice

1 tablespoon Asian fish sauce

½ teaspoon sugar

1 green Thai chili, seeded and minced

2 scallions, diced

2 teaspoons coriander, crushed

½ seedless cucumber, diced

1 teaspoon finely chopped mint leaves

1. Preheat broiler.
2. Broil flank steak strips for 5 minutes on each side.
3. Mix lime juice, fish sauce, sugar, and chili in a bowl.
4. Add the scallions, coriander, cucumber, and steak to the dressing.
5. Arrange on a platter and garnish with mint leaves before serving.

PER SERVING: CALORIES: 151 | FAT: 6G | PROTEIN: 19G | SODIUM: 402MG | FIBER: 1G | CARBOHYDRATES: 4G | SUGAR: 2G

TAKE NOTE

Mint makes a good herb garden staple. It can be used to add zip to bland recipes and garnish everything from desserts to salads. Mint leaves have been used as a garnish since the early 1920s because they add an irresistible zest to a variety of flavors. They are also used to garnish cocktails.

HOLLYWOOD LOBSTER SALAD
YIELDS 4 SERVINGS

¾ pound lobster meat, cooked and torn into chunks

4 tablespoons extra-virgin olive oil

1 teaspoon lemon juice

3 tablespoons chopped chives

⅓ cup fat-free Miracle Whip salad dressing

Salt and pepper, to taste

1 head Boston lettuce, rinsed and torn

1. Gently fold all ingredients except the lettuce together.
2. Cover and refrigerate until chilled.
3. Arrange lobster mixture on a bed of lettuce and serve immediately.

PER SERVING: CALORIES: 250 | FAT: 16G | PROTEIN: 23G | SODIUM: 214MG | FIBER: 1G | CARBOHYDRATES: 4G | SUGAR: 1G

▶ ENTRÉES

BEEF FAJITAS

YIELDS 4 SERVINGS

1 pound extra-lean beef round steaks, cut into thin strips

1 envelope fajita seasoning mix

1 small onion, diced

1 green bell pepper, sliced

1 small red bell pepper, sliced

½ cup water

1 (11-ounce) package corn tortillas

1. Sprinkle steak strips with fajita seasoning in a medium bowl, making sure to cover all sides.
2. Sauté onion and peppers in heavy skillet over medium heat until soft.
3. Add steak to vegetables and add water.
4. Cover and simmer over low heat for 3–4 hours, stirring occasionally.
5. Serve with tortillas (or over rice).

PER SERVING: CALORIES: 492 | FAT: 16G | PROTEIN: 42G | SODIUM: 786MG | FIBER: 6G | CARBOHYDRATES: 46G | SUGAR: 5G

TAKE NOTE

When you sauté multiple ingredients and liquids on the stove, you need to make sure you use a skillet or frying pan with high sides, at least about 1½", to minimize splatter. A splatter screen is also a good investment. Not only does splattered oil make a mess of your stovetop and clothes; it hurts when it hits your skin!

GARLIC PORK LOIN
YIELDS 4 SERVINGS

1 packet dry onion soup mix

2 pounds pork roast, fat removed

1 teaspoon fresh rosemary

2 garlic cloves, crushed

1 teaspoon dry mustard

1 teaspoon marjoram leaves

1. Preheat oven to 300°F. Line a shallow baking pan with heavy-duty aluminum foil.
2. Sprinkle onion soup mix on the bottom of the pan. Place roast on top of soup mix. Sprinkle rosemary, garlic, mustard, and marjoram on top of roast. Cover roast with aluminum foil.
3. Bake for 3½–4 hours or until completely done.

PER SERVING: CALORIES: 322 | FAT: 9G | PROTEIN: 51G | SODIUM: 915MG | FIBER: 1G | CARBOHYDRATES: 7G | SUGAR: 1G

ZESTY CRUMB-COATED COD
YIELDS 3 SERVINGS

1 lemon

1 slice whole-wheat bread

1 pound cod fillet

Salt and pepper, to taste

1. Preheat the broiler.
2. Squeeze 2 tablespoons of lemon juice into a food processor. Place bread in the food processor and pulse until crumbs form.
3. Place cod in a baking pan and squeeze remaining lemon juice over, to your liking. Sprinkle cod with salt and pepper. Pat cod fillet with the bread crumbs, turning fillet so you get both sides.
4. Broil for about 8 minutes or until crumbs turn golden.

PER SERVING: CALORIES: 163 | FAT: 2G | PROTEIN: 28G | SODIUM: 142MG | FIBER: 1G | CARBOHYDRATES: 7G | SUGAR: 1G

SHRIMP AND CHICKEN JAMBALAYA

YIELDS 4 SERVINGS

1 tablespoon olive oil

1 onion, chopped

3 cloves garlic, minced

1 red pepper, chopped

1 green pepper, chopped

1 (16-ounce) can chopped tomatoes, with juice

3 cups low-sodium chicken broth

1 teaspoon dried thyme

1 teaspoon dried basil

⅛ teaspoon cayenne pepper

⅛ teaspoon ground cloves

⅛ teaspoon ground allspice

¾ cup long-grain rice

1 pound shrimp, deveined and peeled

2 chicken breast fillets, sliced in thin strips

2 tablespoons chopped fresh parsley

1. Heat olive oil in a large skillet over medium heat. Add the onion, garlic, and peppers. Stir until the onions begin to soften, adding a spoonful or two of water if necessary to keep the mixture from sticking.
2. Stir in the tomatoes, chicken broth, thyme, basil, cayenne, cloves, and allspice. Bring to a boil over high heat, reduce heat to medium, and simmer for 5 minutes.
3. Stir in the rice. Return to a boil over high heat, reduce heat to medium, and cover.
4. Cook for 20 minutes, then add the shrimp, chicken, and parsley.
5. Simmer until the rice is done and the shrimp and chicken are cooked. Serve immediately.

PER SERVING: CALORIES: 462 | FAT: 8G | PROTEIN: 55G | SODIUM: 507MG | FIBER: 4G | CARBOHYDRATES: 41G | SUGAR: 8G

CHICKEN MARSALA
YIELDS 4 SERVINGS

Salt and pepper, to taste

1 cup flour

4 (4-ounce) skinless, boneless chicken breasts

¼ cup canola oil

3–4 slices prosciutto ham, thinly sliced

½ cup sliced porcini mushrooms

½ cup sweet Marsala wine

½ cup chicken stock

2 tablespoons unsalted butter

½ cup flat-leaf parsley

1. Mix salt and pepper in flour.
2. Dredge chicken breasts in flour.
3. Heat canola oil in large pan over medium heat.
4. Fry chicken on both sides until brown, about 5 minutes for each side.
5. Remove chicken from pan. Add ham to the skillet and sauté for 1 minute.
6. Take out ham and sauté mushrooms until they are brown and dry.
7. Pour Marsala wine into the pan to boil down, about 10 seconds.
8. Add chicken stock and simmer for a minute.
9. Stir in butter and add chicken and ham.
10. Simmer until chicken is heated through.
11. Season to taste and garnish with parsley before serving.

PER SERVING: CALORIES: 540 | FAT: 26G | PROTEIN: 37G | SODIUM: 951MG | FIBER: 2G | CARBOHYDRATES: 30G | SUGAR: 1G

TURKEY CASSEROLE

YIELDS 4 SERVINGS

3 cups cooked light-meat turkey

1 (8-ounce) can pineapple chunks, drained

½ cup apricot preserves

1 (10-ounce) can cream of chicken soup

1 (8-ounce) can sliced water chestnuts

⅓ cup water

2 cups cooked rice

1. Preheat oven to 350°F.
2. Mix all ingredients in a large bowl.
3. Place ingredients in a lightly greased cooking dish.
4. Bake uncovered for 35 minutes. Serve immediately.

PER SERVING: CALORIES: 473 | FAT: 4G | PROTEIN: 36G | SODIUM: 364MG | FIBER: 3G | CARBOHYDRATES: 73G | SUGAR: 28G

TAKE NOTE

Casseroles date back to the early eighteenth century when meat was slowly cooked in clay containers with rice. Today you can bake them in the oven, and they can be ready in less than an hour. You can also adapt your recipe for an easy slow-cooker meal.

VEGETABLE STUFFED PEPPERS

YIELDS 4 SERVINGS

4 green bell peppers

6 cups water

1 (15-ounce) can pinto beans, rinsed and drained

2 cups whole-kernel corn

¾ cup low-fat shredded cheddar cheese

½ tablespoon vegetable oil

1 clove garlic, crushed

½ onion, chopped

1 teaspoon black pepper

1. Preheat oven to 375°F.
2. Cut off the tops of the green peppers. Remove the seeds.
3. Boil 6 cups of water; add peppers and cook for 5 minutes. Remove peppers and place upside down on a paper towel to drain.
4. Mix all remaining ingredients in a medium bowl. Divide ingredients evenly among the peppers and stuff them. Place peppers in a baking dish, filled-side up, and bake about 20 minutes. Serve hot.

PER SERVING: CALORIES: 531 | FAT: 11G | PROTEIN: 22G | SODIUM: 441MG | FIBER: 14G | CARBOHYDRATES: 91G | SUGAR: 5G

POLENTA PIE

YIELDS 8 SERVINGS

5 teaspoons olive oil, divided

1 onion, finely chopped

2 (10-ounce) packages frozen chopped spinach, thawed

4 cloves garlic, crushed

Salt and pepper, to taste

3 cups water

3 cups low-sodium vegetable broth

2 cups coarse-ground yellow cornmeal

2 cups tomato sauce, any type

Basil leaves, to garnish

1. Preheat oven to 375°F. Use 1 teaspoon of olive oil to lightly oil a ceramic quiche dish; set aside.
2. Heat 3 teaspoons of oil in a large skillet over medium heat. Add the onion and sauté for about 2 minutes. Add the thawed spinach; sauté until soft. Add the garlic, salt, and pepper; continue to stir for 5 minutes, then set aside.
3. Combine the water, broth, and cornmeal in a medium bowl.
4. Spoon half of the polenta into the quiche dish, pressing it down with your fingers or the back of a spoon to make a smooth surface. Spoon in the spinach filling, spreading evenly. Spoon remaining polenta over spinach, spreading evenly. Brush top of polenta layer with remaining teaspoon of oil.
5. Cover with foil and bake for 30 minutes; then remove the foil and bake for another 15 minutes, or until the top is browned. Remove from oven, top each serving with tomato sauce and basil, and serve while hot.

PER SERVING: CALORIES: 196 | FAT: 4G | PROTEIN: 5G | SODIUM: 639MG | FIBER: 5G | CARBOHYDRATES: 36G | SUGAR: 5G

PASTA CARBONARA

YIELDS 6 SERVINGS

1 pound spaghetti

½ cup Egg Beaters

¼ cup grated Parmesan cheese

¼ cup grated Pecorino-Romano cheese

Morton's lite salt, to taste

Cracked pepper, to taste

½ cup diced pancetta

1. Cook spaghetti according to package directions.
2. In a large mixing bowl, whisk the Egg Beaters, Parmesan, Pecorino, salt, and pepper until it is thick and creamy.
3. Mix the egg mixture and pasta together carefully.
4. Add the pancetta. Serve hot.

PER SERVING: CALORIES: 358 | FAT: 6G | PROTEIN: 16G | SODIUM: 330MG | FIBER: 2G | CARBOHYDRATES: 57G | SUGAR: 2G

TAKE NOTE

It is important to make sure the pasta is very hot when added to the egg mixture because it blends better with the pasta to make a creamy coating. If the pasta is not hot enough, the sauce will appear chunky.

MACARONI AND CHEESE
YIELDS 4 SERVINGS

2 cups macaroni noodles

½ stalk celery, minced

¼ cup minced onion

2 tablespoons canola oil

3 tablespoons fat-free milk

4 tablespoons flour

1 cup low-fat grated cheddar cheese

½ cup low-fat grated Swiss cheese

½ teaspoon grated nutmeg

Salt and pepper, to taste

1. Cook macaroni according to package directions.
2. Sauté minced celery and onion in a skillet with the oil over medium heat.
3. Mix in the milk and flour, stirring until smooth.
4. Mix in the cheese, stirring constantly until thick.
5. Remove immediately from heat.
6. Stir in the nutmeg and season with salt and pepper.
7. Pour mixture over the macaroni. Toss and serve.

PER SERVING: CALORIES: 366 | FAT: 10G | PROTEIN: 19G | SODIUM: 221MG | FIBER: 2G | CARBOHYDRATES: 48G | SUGAR: 3G

TAKE NOTE
Nutmeg always adds a slight hint of spice and helps bring out the flavor in cheese sauces. You can use a pinch of ground nutmeg, but freshly-ground nutmeg has much more flavor and aroma. Keep a whole nutmeg in a tiny grater made just for that purpose, and grate a bit of fresh nutmeg over everything from cheese sauce to potatoes.

▶ DESSERTS

CHEESECAKE
YIELDS 8 SERVINGS

1 cup finely crushed reduced-fat
graham crackers

¼ cup butter, melted

16 ounces fat-free cream cheese

½ cup sugar

1 teaspoon vanilla

2 egg whites

3 tablespoons cake flour

¼ teaspoon salt

½ cup fat-free milk

1. Preheat oven to 350°F.
2. Stir the graham-cracker crumbs and butter together until they are evenly mixed.
3. Press crumb mixture into the bottom of a baking pan.
4. Mix cream cheese, sugar, vanilla, and egg whites in a medium bowl with an electric mixer until cream cheese is fluffy.
5. Add the cake flour, salt, and milk. Mix thoroughly.
6. Pour batter into the crust. Bake for 1 hour.
7. Cool before placing in fridge.
8. Refrigerate at least 3 hours before serving.

PER SERVING: CALORIES: 228 | FAT: 7G | PROTEIN: 11G | SODIUM: 586MG | FIBER: 1G | CARBOHYDRATES: 29G | SUGAR: 19G

TAKE NOTE
To safely freeze a cheesecake, place it in the freezer uncovered until it is frozen through. Tightly wrap the cheesecake in two layers of plastic wrap and cover with aluminum foil. Do not keep the cheesecake frozen for longer than a month. When you are ready to eat the cheesecake, thaw it out by removing it to the refrigerator overnight.

BUTTERSCOTCH CUPCAKES

YIELDS 16 SERVINGS

½ cup cake flour

¾ cup powdered sugar

5 egg whites

⅛ teaspoon salt

1 teaspoon heavy cream

½ cup butterscotch ice cream topping

¼ cup granulated sugar

½ teaspoon vanilla

1. Preheat oven to 350°F.
2. Line muffin tins with cupcake liners and set aside.
3. In a large bowl, sift the cake flour and powdered sugar twice.
4. In a medium bowl, beat the egg whites and salt with an electric mixer until frothy.
5. Add heavy cream and butterscotch, beating until soft peaks form.
6. Add sugar and continue beating until well combined.
7. Fold in flour mixture gradually until blended.
8. Add vanilla. Mix thoroughly.
9. Spoon batter into muffin cups.
10. Bake for 20 minutes or until cupcake tops are browned.

PER SERVING: CALORIES: 82 | FAT: 0G | PROTEIN: 2G | SODIUM: 72MG | FIBER: 0G | CARBOHYDRATES: 19G | SUGAR: 9G

APPLESAUCE-SOUR CREAM COFFEE CAKE

YIELDS 20 SERVINGS

Light cooking spray

1½ cups flour

¾ cup packed light brown sugar

1 teaspoon baking soda

½ teaspoon baking powder

1 teaspoon ground cinnamon

1 teaspoon salt

¾ cup fat-free sour cream

2 tablespoons canola oil

1 cup unsweetened applesauce

1. Preheat oven to 350°F.
2. Coat a square baking pan with light cooking spray.
3. Mix the flour, brown sugar, baking soda, baking powder, cinnamon, and salt in a large bowl.
4. Mix the sour cream, oil, and applesauce in a small bowl.
5. Add sour cream mixture to flour mixture. Mix well but do not beat.
6. Pour batter into baking pan and bake until done, about 40 minutes.

PER SERVING: CALORIES: 92 | FAT: 2G | PROTEIN: 1G | SODIUM: 203MG | FIBER: 0G | CARBOHYDRATES: 18G | SUGAR: 10G

MANGO ANGEL FLUFF

YIELDS 12 SERVINGS

4 pasteurized egg whites

1 cup sugar

1 tablespoon lemon juice

7½ ounces frozen mangoes, thawed

1 cup heavy whipping cream

2 tablespoons powdered sugar

1 teaspoon vanilla

1 cup flaked coconut

1. Place egg whites in a large bowl; let stand for 30 minutes at room temperature. Add sugar, lemon juice, and mangoes. Beat with a hand mixer until combined; then beat for 15 minutes at high speed, until mixture is thick and triples in volume.

2. In a medium bowl, beat whipping cream with powdered sugar and vanilla until stiff. Fold into meringue along with coconut. Rinse a 10" ring mold with water and shake out over sink; do not dry mold. Pour coconut mixture into mold. Cover and freeze until firm.

3. To unmold, rinse a kitchen towel in hot water and wring out. Place mold on serving plate. Drape hot towel over mold for 10–15 seconds to loosen dessert. Remove mold, let stand at room temperature for 15 minutes, slice, and serve with raspberry sauce.

PER SERVING: CALORIES: 128 | FAT: 10G | PROTEIN: 2G | SODIUM 28MG | FIBER: 1G | CARBOHYDRATES: 22G | SUGAR: 21G

TAKE NOTE

When recipes call for raw eggs, you should consider using pasteurized eggs. They are more expensive but worth it. Be sure to watch the expiration date on these eggs and discard them after that date has passed. It does take longer for pasteurized whites to whip, but just keep working; they will fluff up.

LEMON PIE
YIELDS 12 SERVINGS

Zest and juice of 2 lemons

½ cup Egg Beaters

½ cup sugar

4 pasteurized egg whites

4 cups light Cool Whip

5½ ounces vanilla wafer cookies

1. Squeeze the lemons to get ½ cup juice.
2. In a double boiler, cook the Egg Beaters, sugar, and lemon juice over simmering water until it gets thick.
3. Remove from heat and stir in the lemon zest.
4. Pour entire mixture into a medium bowl and put in refrigerator until it is cold.
5. Whip the egg whites to form stiff peaks.
6. Mix about ⅓ of the egg whites into the cold lemon mixture.
7. Fold in the rest of the whites and the Cool Whip topping until it is all well blended.
8. Crush the vanilla wafers in a freezer bag.
9. Line two pie tins with vanilla wafer crumbs, saving some to sprinkle over the tops of the pies.
10. Fill the pie tins with the lemon mixture. Sprinkle the remaining crumbs over the tops. Place the pies in the freezer until firm.
11. Remove from the freezer about 10 minutes before you plan to serve to slightly thaw and make it easier to slice.

PER SERVING: CALORIES: 158 | FAT: 5G | PROTEIN: 3G | SODIUM: 88MG | FIBER: 0G | CARBOHYDRATES: 27G | SUGAR: 16G

PUMPKIN PIE
YIELDS 12 SERVINGS

¾ cup packed brown sugar

¼ teaspoon salt

2 teaspoons cinnamon

1 tablespoon nutmeg

12 ounces evaporated low-fat milk

2 egg whites

1 whole egg

15 ounces unsweetened pumpkin

Light cooking spray

8 ounces packaged pie dough

1. Preheat oven to 425°F.
2. Mix the brown sugar, salt, cinnamon, nutmeg, evaporated milk, egg whites, whole egg, and pumpkin in a large bowl. Stir with a whisk and set aside.
3. Spray pie pan with the light cooking spray.
4. Press the dough into the pie pan, covering the bottom and all sides.
5. Pour the pie mixture into the pie pan.
6. Bake for 50 minutes. Serve warm.

PER SERVING: CALORIES: 188 | FAT: 7G | PROTEIN: 5G | SODIUM: 194MG | FIBER: 2G | CARBOHYDRATES: 28G | SUGAR: 18G

TAKE NOTE
When a recipe calls for canned pumpkin, be sure you buy and use what is called "solid pack" pumpkin. If you use canned pumpkin-pie filling, the recipe will fail because that ingredient contains sugar, emulsifiers, and liquids in addition to pumpkin. If you're feeling ambitious, you could cook and purée a fresh pumpkin and use that.

APPLE PIE

YIELDS 10 SERVINGS

2 cups plus 3 tablespoons all-purpose flour, divided

6 tablespoons ice water

1 teaspoon apple cider vinegar

2 tablespoons powdered sugar

1½ teaspoons salt, divided

7 tablespoons vegetable shortening

8 cups peeled and thinly sliced Granny Smith apples

1 tablespoon fresh lemon juice

⅔ cup plus 1 tablespoon sugar, divided

1 teaspoon cinnamon

1 teaspoon ground nutmeg

1 egg white

1. Combine ½ cup flour, ice water, and vinegar, stirring with a whisk until well blended.
2. Mix in 1½ cups flour, powdered sugar, and ½ teaspoon salt in a large bowl.
3. Mix in shortening with two knives until mixture resembles coarse meal.
4. Divide dough in half.
5. Gently press each half into a 4" circle on two sheets of overlapping heavy-duty plastic wrap; cover with two additional sheets of overlapping plastic wrap.
6. Roll one dough half, still covered, into a 12" circle. Repeat with the other half.
7. Chill dough for 10 minutes or until plastic wrap can be easily removed.
8. Preheat oven to 375°F, then prepare filling by combining the apples and lemon juice in a large bowl.
9. Mix ⅔ cup sugar, 3 tablespoons flour, cinnamon, nutmeg, and ⅛ teaspoon salt in a small bowl.
10. Sprinkle sugar mixture over apples and toss well to coat.
11. Lightly spray pie plates with cooking spray.

12. Remove top two sheets of plastic wrap from one 12" dough circle. Fit dough, plastic wrap–side up, into the pie plate, allowing dough to extend over edge.

13. Remove remaining plastic wrap. Spoon filling into dough; brush edges of dough lightly with water.

14. Remove top two sheets of plastic wrap from the remaining dough circle; place, plastic wrap–side up, on top of filled pie plate. Remove remaining plastic wrap. Press edges of dough together. Fold edges under. Cut several 1" slits in top of pastry using a sharp knife.

15. Brush top and edges of pie with egg white; sprinkle with 1 tablespoon sugar.

16. Bake for 40 minutes or until top is golden brown. Chill well before serving.

PER SERVING: CALORIES: 287 | FAT: 9G | PROTEIN: 3G | SODIUM: 360MG | FIBER: 2G | CARBOHYDRATES: 49G | SUGAR: 25G

CLASSIC OATMEAL COOKIES

YIELDS 24 SERVINGS

Light cooking spray

1 cup sugar

¼ cup margarine, softened

2 eggs

¾ cup unsweetened applesauce

1 teaspoon vanilla

2 cups flour

½ teaspoon baking soda

¼ teaspoon salt

1 cup uncooked oats

1. Preheat oven to 375°F.
2. Prepare baking sheets with light cooking spray. Set aside.
3. Beat the sugar and margarine in a large bowl with a hand mixer.
4. Add the eggs, applesauce, and vanilla, mixing well.
5. Combine flour, baking soda, and salt in a medium bowl.
6. Add flour mixture to sugar mixture. Beat well.
7. Stir in the oats and mix well.
8. Drop dough into mounds on baking sheets, about 2" apart.
9. Bake for 15 minutes or until cookies are golden brown.

PER SERVING: CALORIES: 122 | FAT: 3G | PROTEIN: 3G | SODIUM: 57MG |
FIBER: 1G | CARBOHYDRATES: 22G | SUGAR: 9G

CRISP ICEBOX COOKIES

YIELDS 48 SERVINGS

¾ cup butter, softened

¼ cup coconut oil

1 cup brown sugar

1 cup sugar

2 eggs

2 teaspoons vanilla

2¼ cups flour

1 teaspoon baking soda

½ teaspoon salt

1 cup finely chopped cashews

1. In a large bowl, beat butter and coconut oil until blended. Gradually add brown sugar and sugar; beat until fluffy. Add eggs and vanilla and mix well. Stir in flour, baking soda, and salt.
2. Shape dough into three long rolls, about 1½" in diameter. Roll the cookie rolls in the chopped cashews, gently pressing nuts into dough to adhere. Wrap well in wax paper, then put rolls into plastic food-storage bags. Chill for at least 24 hours.
3. Preheat oven to 375°F. Cut the dough into slices about ¼" thick and place on ungreased baking sheets. Bake for 6–8 minutes or until cookies are set and very light golden brown. Cool on cookie sheets for 3 minutes, then remove to wire racks to cool completely.

PER SERVING: CALORIES: 110 | FAT: 6G | PROTEIN: 1G | SODIUM: 74MG | FIBER: 0G | CARBOHYDRATES: 14G | SUGAR: 9G

TAKE NOTE

If you're pressed for time, these icebox cookies are a great choice. You can make the dough one day, then chill it in the refrigerator and bake the next day, or the next. This cookie dough also freezes very well. Wrap the dough rolls in freezer wrap and place them in freezer plastic bags. You can slice and bake the dough from frozen; just add a few minutes to the baking time.

SUGAR COOKIES
YIELDS 20 SERVINGS

1 cup flour

½ cup whole-wheat flour

¾ cup sugar

¼ teaspoon salt

1 teaspoon baking powder

3 tablespoons canola oil

1 egg

2 tablespoons skim milk

2 teaspoons vanilla

Light cooking spray

1. Preheat oven to 350°F.
2. Mix all dry ingredients in a large bowl.
3. Mix all liquid ingredients in a medium bowl; add to dry ingredients and mix thoroughly.
4. Spray baking sheets with light cooking spray.
5. Drop cookie dough balls about 2" apart on baking sheets.
6. Bake for 8–10 minutes or until slightly browned on edges.

PER SERVING: CALORIES: 84 | FAT: 2G | PROTEIN: 1G | SODIUM: 58MG | FIBER: 0G | CARBOHYDRATES: 15G | SUGAR: 8G

AFTERWORD

While tapping therapies were originally designed to focus on the emotional problems you are struggling with, and to release the emotional and energetic conflict stored in your energy system, many people have put more of a positive spin on tapping in recent years. Sometimes they use positive wording in subsequent rounds after a few sequences of focusing on the problem. We could call this more positive approach "Thank-You Tapping."

▶ THANK-YOU TAPPING

I started using Thank-You Tapping as part of my plan for gratitude and giving thanks for what I have in my life, and it is now hugely popular in the EFT field.

Start with Regular Tapping

You start by following the same five-step method as before.

Step 1. Choose a target. For example, perhaps it is "I feel stress in my life."

Step 2. Measure your level of stress on the 0–10 point scale.

Step 3. Create your setup statement, such as, "Even though I feel stress and worry in my life, I deeply and completely love and accept myself."

Step 4. Start tapping. Begin by tapping the karate chop point while saying your setup statement. Repeat three times. Then move through the sequence of acupuncture points.

1. *Eyebrow: I feel stress in my life.*
2. *Side of Eye: I feel stress in my body and mind.*

3. *Under Eye: I don't know how to calm down.*
4. *Under Nose: I feel a lot of stress in my life.*
5. *Chin: I don't know how to feel better.*
6. *Collarbone: All this stress in my life.*
7. *Under Arm: I feel the stress and tension building up.*
8. *Head: I feel all this stress and tension.*

Step 5. Measure your level of distress again. Take a deep breath, and consider the level of stress you feel again on the 0–10 point scale. You can do one more round of tapping on your stress level and focus on what you're worried about, and then you can switch to Thank-You Tapping.

End with Thank-You Tapping

For a subsequent round of tapping, focus on gratitude and thankfulness in your rephrased statements. For example, you might try wording like this:

1. *Eyebrow: Thank you, Universe, for bringing me so much success in my life.*
2. *Side of Eye: Thank You, Divine Intelligence, for bringing me a resolution to that work problem.*
3. *Under Eye: Thank you, Universe, for so much love in my life.*
4. *Under Nose: Thank you, Universe, for ease around my eating issues.*
5. *Chin: Thank you, Universe, for bringing me peace in my life.*
6. *Collarbone: Thank you, Universe, for bringing me contentment.*
7. *Under Arm: Thank you, Universe, for the time to reflect on my feelings.*
8. *Head: Thank you, Universe, for bringing me so much peace in my life.*

Take a deep breath, and enjoy the positive feelings in your body and mind. You can repeat rounds of tapping while saying "Thank You, Universe (or God or Higher Power or Nature)," or you can focus on one particular topic of health, weight, relationships, or confidence.

U.S./METRIC CONVERSION CHART

VOLUME CONVERSIONS

U.S. Volume Measure	Metric Equivalent
⅛ teaspoon	0.5 milliliter
¼ teaspoon	1 milliliter
½ teaspoon	2 milliliters
1 teaspoon	5 milliliters
½ tablespoon	7 milliliters
1 tablespoon (3 teaspoons)	15 milliliters
2 tablespoons (1 fluid ounce)	30 milliliters
¼ cup (4 tablespoons)	60 milliliters
⅓ cup	90 milliliters
½ cup (4 fluid ounces)	125 milliliters
⅔ cup	160 milliliters
¾ cup (6 fluid ounces)	180 milliliters
1 cup (16 tablespoons)	250 milliliters
1 pint (2 cups)	500 milliliters
1 quart (4 cups)	1 liter (about)

WEIGHT CONVERSIONS

U.S. Weight Measure	Metric Equivalent
½ ounce	15 grams
1 ounce	30 grams
2 ounces	60 grams
3 ounces	85 grams
¼ pound (4 ounces)	115 grams
½ pound (8 ounces)	225 grams
¾ pound (12 ounces)	340 grams
1 pound (16 ounces)	454 grams

U.S./METRIC CONVERSION CHART

OVEN TEMPERATURE CONVERSIONS	
Degrees Fahrenheit	*Degrees Celsius*
200 degrees F	95 degrees C
250 degrees F	120 degrees C
275 degrees F	135 degrees C
300 degrees F	150 degrees C
325 degrees F	160 degrees C
350 degrees F	180 degrees C
375 degrees F	190 degrees C
400 degrees F	205 degrees C
425 degrees F	220 degrees C
450 degrees F	230 degrees C

BAKING PAN SIZES	
U.S.	*Metric*
8 × 1½ inch round baking pan	20 × 4 cm cake tin
9 × 1½ inch round baking pan	23 × 3.5 cm cake tin
11 × 7 × 1½ inch baking pan	28 × 18 × 4 cm baking tin
13 × 9 × 2 inch baking pan	30 × 20 × 5 cm baking tin
2 quart rectangular baking dish	30 × 20 × 3 cm baking tin
15 × 10 × 2 inch baking pan	30 × 25 × 2 cm baking tin (Swiss roll tin)
9 inch pie plate	22 × 4 or 23 × 4 cm pie plate
7 or 8 inch springform pan	18 or 20 cm springform or loose-bottom cake tin
9 × 5 × 3 inch loaf pan	23 × 13 × 7 cm or 2 lb narrow loaf or pâté tin
1½ quart casserole	1.5 liter casserole
2 quart casserole	2 liter casserole

INDEX

Heat, point on top of, 23
Hollywood Lobster Salad, 202
Honey and Cheese-Stuffed Figs, 186
Hot Crab Dip, 192
Hunger
  emotional, 29
  for non-food things, 28–31
  physical, 29
  setup statements for, 73–74
  spiritual, 29–30
Hurt, setup statements for, 74
Hurt, tapping on (scripts), 128–30

Icebox cookies, 222
Identity and safety issues, 43–45
Insecurity, setup statements for, 78–80

Jambalaya, shrimp and chicken, 206
Journal writing, 106–7

Late-evening script, 100–102
Lemon Pie, 217
Logic, limits of, 34–35
Loneliness, setup statements for, 75–76
Loneliness, tapping on (scripts), 127–28
Love, hunger for, 19, 28
Low-Fat Egg and Spinach Cupcakes, 174

Macaroni and Cheese, 212
Mango Angel Fluff, 216
Marinara Dip, 188
Measurement conversion chart, 227–28
Measuring distress level, 20, 23, 67–69, 84
Meditation, 109–11
  basic steps, 109–10
  benefits of, 109
  mindfulness and, 107–8, 109
  script, 110–11
  visualization and, 111–13
Memories of past experiences, target

Meridians, 14, 18
Mifflin-St. Jeor equation, 151–52
Mindfulness, 107–8
Morning script, 89–92
Muffins. *See* Breads

Noon script, 92–94
Nose, point under, 22
Nutmeg, about, 212
Nuts
  about: daily intake, 165; fats in, 165; as superfood/nutritional benefits, 164–65; types of, 165
  Triple-Play Chocolate–Banana Nut Muffins, 181

Oatmeal Banana Bread, 178
Oatmeal cookies. *See also* Corn
Omega-3 fatty acids, 157–58, 163, 164
Overeating
  case study, 17–18
  emotional core of, 28–31
  how tapping helps, 17–18
  as symptom of real problem, 32–33

Pasta
  Macaroni and Cheese, 212
  Pasta Carbonara, 211
Pear and Watercress Salad, 199
Peppers, vegetable stuffed, 209
Physical, hunger for, 29
Physical symptoms, targeting examples, 66–67
Pies. *See* Desserts
Plan. *See* Daily plan
Plateaus
  setup statements for, 76
  tapping for, 60
Polenta Pie, 210
Pork
  Eggs Benedict, 176
  Garlic Pork Loin, 204

ABOUT THE AUTHORS

Carol Look has been a pioneer in the EFT community for more than seventeen years. Combining her background as a traditional psychotherapist with energy psychology, Look is a premier success and abundance coach, inspiring people to attract abundance into their lives by using EFT. She has been a popular guest on the industry's leading Healing Telesummits, such as *The Tapping Solution*, which reaches more than 1 million listeners. She is respected around the globe as a dynamic international speaker, and has taught EFT workshops at prestigious organizations like Kripalu, Omega Institute, and the Association for Comprehensive Energy Psychology. She runs a successful coaching program and mentors practitioners worldwide. For more on Carol, please visit *www.CarolLook.com*.

Jill Cerreta is a registered dietitian and nutrition consultant. In 2011, she started Live Well Nutrition, and also works as a consultant for *Eating Well* magazine. She lives in Vermont with her family.